"We are only just now coming to recognize a truth that should have been apparent for a long time. The control of excess body weight is a lifetime problem which requires a lifetime commitment. Our preoccupation with the short-term perspective of the latest reducing diet has for too long obscured this painful truth.

"Dr. Kirschenbaum's new book is important in recognizing the nature of the problem and in preparing the overweight person to cope with it. It provides no fancy diets or easy fixes but makes clear what is necessary for long-term weight control. He begins with a convincing explanation of why there is a problem, describing in a succinct manner the power of biology to determine our body weight. Once these biological determinants have become clear, it is apparent why a lifelong change in lifestyle is necessary. Dr. Kirschenbaum uses his rich clinical experience in the treatment of obesity to present a sane and sensible program of lifestyle change. An important *leitmotiv* of this program is the need for continuing effort, a theme well conveyed by the title, *Weight Loss Through Persistence*. Written in a lively and engaging style, this volume illustrates the latest approach to the control of body weight. It deserves widespread attention."

—Albert J. Stunkard, M.D., Professor of Psychiatry,
    University of Pennsylvania School of Medicine

"*Weight Loss Through Persistence* effectively combines scientifically proven procedures for losing weight and keeping it off with a clear, readable portrayal of the common pitfalls along the way. Beginning with a discussion of common myths and misconceptions, the book provides a lucid and informative exposition of Dr. Kirschenbaum's own research on the stages of change in weight control which he then uses as a framework for readers to develop persistence in the pursuit of nutritional, exercise, and broader lifestyle goals. Throughout the book the emphasis on persistence is repeatedly coupled with a variety of tasks that will surely captivate the reader and offer the motivation to negotiate the myriad of difficulties in achieving weight control. Special features of the book are the inclusion of many examples from Dr. Kirschenbaum's clients that nicely illustrate the key points, nutritious recipes, and a very important chapter on coping with stress."

—William G. Johnson, Ph.D., Professor of Psychiatry,
    University of Mississippi Medical Center

"Dr. Kirschenbaum has created a self-help *tour de force* for anyone interested in controlling his or her weight. This book will replace at least one hundred handouts used in our weight control program. This master scientist and clinician offers hope, guidance, and encouragement for individuals who want to apply the latest scientific knowledge in order to maintain persistence on their difficult journey. Our patients will greatly benefit from this book!"

—Raymond C. Baker, Ph.D., St. Francis Medical Center, Peoria, Illinois

"Finally, everyone can now benefit from the summation of more than 20 years of scientific research and clinical experience in the treatment of obesity by an internationally acknowledged expert. I know my patients will be thankful."

—Randall C. Flanery, Ph.D., Director, Eating Disorders Program, Division of Behavioral Medicine, St. Louis University Health Sciences Center

"Four stars for readability, completeness, and compassion. This will be our treatment manual for many years to come."

—Kimberly A. Chupurdia, Ph.D., Baltimore, Maryland

"Professor Kirschenbaum's masterful approach has influenced hundreds of behavioral scientists. It's the truth, the whole truth; read it, memorize it, use it."

—Eileen H. Rosendahl, Ph.D., Albert Einstein College of Medicine

# Weight Loss Through Persistence

## Making Science Work for You

DANIEL S. KIRSCHENBAUM, Ph.D.

NEW HARBINGER PUBLICATIONS, INC.

## Publisher's Note

This publication is designed to provide accurate and authoritative information in regard to the subject matter covered. It is sold with the understanding that the publisher is not engaged in rendering psychological, financial, legal, or other professional services. If expert assistance or counseling is needed, the services of a competent professional should be sought.

Many of the designations used by manufacturers and sellers to distinguish their products are claimed as trademarks. Where those designations appear in this book and New Harbinger Publications was aware of a trademark claim, the designations have been printed in initial capital letters (e.g., Weight Watchers).

Distributed in the U.S.A. primarily by Publishers Group West; in Canada by Raincoast Books; in Great Britain by Airlift Book Company, Ltd.; in South Africa by Real Books, Ltd.; in Australia by Boobook; and in New Zealand by Tandem Press.

Copyright © 1994
Daniel S. Kirschenbaum, Ph.D.
New Harbinger Publications, Inc.
5674 Shattuck Avenue
Oakland, CA 94609

Library of Congress Catalog Card Number: 93-086803
ISBN 1-879237-64-4 Softcover
ISBN 1-879237-65-2 Hardcover

Cover design by SHELBY DESIGNS & ILLUSTRATES
Editor Judith Brown
Text design by Tracy Marie Powell

First printing 1994, 5,000 copies
Second printing September, 1994, 3,000 copies

# Contents

To my clients, for their trust, courage, and instruction about persistence.

# Acknowledgments

This book incorporates knowledge gleaned from working with hundreds of remarkably dedicated clients during the past 21 years. I am indebted to them for allowing me to become a part of their lives and for teaching me so much about courage, grace, commitment, and persistence. My colleagues, particularly Susan Shrifter-Fialkow in recent years, have helped shape the ideas expressed in these pages into their present configuration. I thank the administrators of the Rock Creek Center, Ian Aitken, Jesse Viner, and Elaine Novak, for supporting me and for helping to create the very comfortable place from which this book emerged, the Center for Behavioral Medicine (in Chicago). I am also most appreciative of Ronnie Rickhoff's mastery of manuscript preparation and Judith Brown's gracious expertise as a copy editor.

Sincere thanks also go to New Harbinger's owners Matt McKay and Pat Fanning, and their staff, for their infectious enthusiasm and professionalism. I was also most fortunate to have Sheila Macomber collaborating with me to create the illustrations in this book; she plays her sophisticated computer graphics program like a Stradivarius.

Finally, the affection and encouragement of my psychologist wife, Laura Humphrey (who helped create the title for this book and who has consistently expanded my perspectives) and the unbridled inspirational curiosity and creativity of our children, Alex and Max, provided considerable energy for this work.

# 1

# Beginning

### Persistence

Nothing in the world can take the place of persistence.
Talent will not;
nothing is more common than unsuccessful people
with talent.
Genius will not;
unrewarded genius is almost a proverb.
Education will not;
the world is full of educated derelicts.
Persistence and determination alone are omnipotent.

—Calvin Coolidge, 1932

All successful weight controllers persist. They persist in spite of their bodies' seemingly insatiable desire to eat. They exercise despite the usual excuses of time, effort, money, and aches and pains. They persist even though they live in a sea of Mrs. Field's cookies and an age of motorized dessert carts. They even persist after a vacation full of deviations or a holiday full of unresisted temptations, and after several very very unwanted pounds have returned—yet again.

You may be wondering, "How can I get myself to do that? Really, *how is that possible?*"

This book *begins* to answer those complicated questions. I have spent 20 years helping people improve their persistence. The ideas in this book have helped me lose 30 pounds and keep it off for 25 years. I have also worked with hundreds of overweight people and many others, such as athletes, who struggle with persistence. Weekend warriors, who take their battles seriously, Olympians, and professional athletes share many of the same concerns that you do. They all struggle to persist in the face of obstacles. They all face obstacles from within themselves, including the limitations of their bodies. They all face obstacles from the competing demands of the rest of their lives: the people and pleasures that take time, the demands of work and school, and the infinite distractions and challenges of life. Yet, the athletes and weight controllers who succeed, like Alice in the following case history, all find ways to persist.

## Case History: Alice Still Lives Here*

Alice turned 48 today. True enough, 48 isn't one of those supposedly especially important birthdays (like 40 or 50), but she often took stock of where she's been and where she's going on her birthdays—whether she was supposed to or not. Alice mentioned to me that she and I have been meeting every week for more than four years now. She recalled her initial enthusiasm for the work we did together and how it helped her harness a lot of energy for weight control. Alice reminded me that she recorded every morsel of food that she ate for many many months in a row back then. Her energized focusing helped her lose more than 40 pounds from her 5-foot-6-inch (initially 240-pound) body in those first six months. After that initial "honeymoon," the struggles became more like swamps than little puddles she used to splash through. Troubles at work, the constant and crazy-making strain of living alone, and other aspects of everyday life began to overtake her efforts to exercise, monitor her eating, and stay focused and optimistic. But, she said, "I never gave up. I came up with new plans almost every week (sometimes almost every day). Sometimes my plans would include new ways of exercising. Can you remember all of the different classes and clubs I joined? Sometimes my plans would stress different types of foods—like my soup plan or my vegetarian plan. I tried Optifast [a liquid meal-replacement approach] about 15 different times over these years: sometimes it helped me lose weight, sometimes the change inspired renewed efforts, sometimes it was just another frustration. But I never gave up, and I never will! I may not get to where I was 30 years ago, but I'm stronger now, healthier, and much thinner than I would be if I did not stay with the struggle every day. [Alice now weighs 60 pounds less and is in much better shape aerobically than she was when she first walked into my office more than four years ago.] I'm learning to live with the struggle. The struggle, and living with it, is okay. At least most of the time it's okay. It's become my roommate! We don't always get along, but we find a way to stay together. It's where I live."

*Note: All of the case materials in this book are based on people whom the author has had the honor of helping during the past 20 years. However, the names and other aspects of each case have been changed to protect the confidentiality of each individual.

## How Do You Become Persistent?

Experience and science provide direction for how to nurture, coax, and otherwise encourage persistence. First, it helps to understand the nature of the obstacles you face. If David did not understand that a well-placed—and well-paced—rock could smite even the biggest man, he would have lost a critical battle that is an inspiration to many. If John F. Kennedy did not appreciate his own charisma, and the fact that television could accentuate this positive quality (especially compared to Richard Nixon), he too would have lost a critical battle. Because you must understand yourself and your foes in order to overcome them, Chapter 2, "Beginning the Battle," describes the nature of the battle for successful weight control and how to begin to win it. "Beginning the Battle" addresses how and why people resist all sorts of changes, not just those made by successful weight controllers. The chapter focuses on the special biological and other challenges faced by weight controllers. When you grasp more fully the challenge of change, you can choose effective goals to guide you toward persistence. In Chapter 2, you will see some examples of goals and how to make strong commitments to them.

Chapter 3, "Stages of Change," looks at expectations. If you expect to fail, you surely will. On the other hand, if you really believe (as many of my clients do at first) that "losing weight is easy," you can also set yourself up to fail. The key questions you can ask are:

What will happen to me during the first two years when I really persist at weight control?

What is it like to pursue this challenge day in and day out for weeks, months, and years?

Research conducted by myself and my co-workers has provided some answers to these important questions. You will learn about the six stages of change that people often experience when attempting to become masterful weight controllers. This idea has helped hundreds of weight controllers clarify their expectations. After reading Chapter 3, you will be able to establish reasonable expectations: *You can expect to succeed if you expect to struggle some of the time and remain committed to persistence all of the time.*

## The Basic Battlegrounds: Eating and Exercising

Chapters 4 and 5 focus on the most basic battlegrounds for weight controllers: eating and exercising. You probably know a great deal about what kind of eating leads to weight loss. Of the hundreds of weight controllers I have had the privilege of helping, almost all of them knew the basics: keep calories low; avoid foods that are high in fats and sugars; diets (highly specific, rigid eating plans) don't work. Chapter 4, "Healthy Eating Ideas," does not belabor these points. However, it reviews the basics and adds a few items that many weight controllers do not appreciate fully. Chapter 5, "Eating Plans," provides some examples of eating plans that work for many successful weight controllers.

Most weight controllers also know that exercising can help them lose weight, but my clients often ask many questions about exercising. For example:

- How much should I exercise?

- Does weight lifting help?

- What types of exercise help the most?

Chapter 6, "Effective Exercising," provides answers to these questions and others.

Also, what if you had your own personal genie who could promise you all the benefits of exercising for the rest of your life if you just wished for it? If you had this wish granted, you would never have to give up sleep again to walk or jog before work, or grind away endless minutes on a treadmill or a stairclimber, or pay another health club bill. Not a bad deal—if only you could get it! Your own willingness (eagerness?) to give up exercising if you could somehow magically get its benefits shows how challenging regular exercising is for almost everybody. The fact is that less than 20 percent of American adults exercise for at least 30 minutes at least twice a week. Successful weight controllers usually exercise almost every day. In other words, *most successful weight controllers exercise more than 95 percent of all Americans.* It takes a powerful commitment to achieve and maintain this level of exercising. Therefore, the discussion of effective exercising focuses on how to become committed to exercise (really committed!) and how to maintain that commitment.

## Taking Control

The first three chapters of the book will help you improve your understanding of the nature of the battle, as well as the battlegrounds of eating and exercising. One point that clearly emerges is:

Becoming a successful weight controller is one of life's most challenging tasks.

The cigarette smoker can give up cigarettes forever. The alcoholic can give up alcohol forever. The medical student or law student can give up time and money for three or four years and then receive a diploma and begin a rewarding career. The athlete can also make many sacrifices but then receive cheers along the way and perhaps a lucrative scholarship, followed by a very lucrative professional salary. Only the weight controller makes sacrifices forever. A few cheers come after the initial weight loss, but then they stop. The effort must continue every day. Weight controllers cannot give up food, and they must maintain a regular exercise program. These challenges do not end after three or four years. They continue throughout life.

A person who has "only" average skills in goal-setting, planning, problem-solving, and self-encouragement will struggle, often unsuccessfully, with the many demands of weight control. *Weight control is so difficult that it requires the use of super-normal personal management skills to achieve success.* The last two chapters of this book may help you improve these skills. I can only say "may help" because these skills do not improve easily. People spend lifetimes developing certain styles of encouraging or discouraging themselves when confronting challenges and certain styles of goal-setting and problem-solving. This book describes methods of goal-setting, planning, and coping that are particularly effective. In Chapter 7, "Taking Control: Improving Self-Control," and Chapter 8, "Stress and Coping," ideas and exercises are presented to help you take the skills you already have to the next level. If you *persist* in working on these skills and make personal development a high priority in your life, you may well begin to manage the demands of weight control more effectively.

## Pathways to Persistence

One central conclusion emerges from the first six chapters: Persistence is the key to successful weight control. You persist more effectively when you understand the challenges you confront, when you make clear commitments to change, and when you know what and how to change. This book includes dozens of ideas and techniques to make all aspects of these pathways to persistence clearer and more attainable.

The final chapter, "Conclusion: Pathways to Persistence," reviews the ideas and techniques presented throughout the book which you can use to improve your persistence at this challenging task. This review can help you develop a lifetime plan for successful weight control. It also discusses when and how to include certain commercial and self-help weight loss programs, professional therapy and programs, and medications in your plan. You may discover, as one of my most successful clients put it, a certain "joy in the discipline." If you do not find much joy in it, you will at least find greater acceptance of the process and yourself. I hope this book helps you make persistence a part of who you are and successful weight control a part of what you accomplish.

# Epilogue

### We Treat Melons Better

When I embark on any new romantic or career venture, there is for me always the same bottom line. Namely, I will assume that, no matter what happens, no matter how deeply I fall in love or how successful the project, if anything goes wrong it is because I prefer buttered rolls to bran flakes for breakfast. Or: I don't have fear of intimacy; my date has a fear of flesh. Okay, maybe I'm exaggerating a little. But the paranoia, the impulse to blame everything on excess tonnage, is undeniably real.

More than anything it's my hope, my fantasy, that someday this horribleness will all go away. Yes, triglycerides are bad, and lack of muscle tone on someone so young is horrendous. But so is such a superficial standard for rating human quality. We treat melons with more dignity. At least we wait to make a judgment until we know what's inside.

—Wendy Wasserstein,
*Bachelor Girls*

# 2

# Beginning the Battle

## The Messages, the Madness

The multibillion-dollar weight loss industry provides a constant barrage of images and slogans, with no regard for your well-being. Think about the underlying messages in slogans like:

- "Lose 22 pounds in one week without dieting and look and feel great."

- "Automatic weight loss: No calorie counting, no hunger pangs, no food restrictions, no painful exercise—guaranteed world's fastest weight loss method."

- "Lose up to 50 pounds or more Without trying! Proven 100% effective—doctor/hospital tested—destroyed existing body fat—helps prevent new fat from forming."

- "Guilt-free, fault-free, fat-free."

- "Now you can eat all you want of these great foods while extra weight disappears: bacon and eggs, roast chicken, roast beef and pork, shrimp, lobster, butter, salad dressings, mayonnaise . . . no self-control needed as 20-30-60-100 unwanted pounds and inches melt away. Absolutely guaranteed amazing results in 2 weeks or a full refund."

One underlying message is: You can lose weight easily and quickly! The before and after photos show just-plain-folks telling you in words and pictures: If I can do it, so can you. Movie stars, politicians, baseball coaches, and disc jockeys echo these messages. Dozens of diet books appear every year full of new twists on old phrases and promises. Here's just a sampling:

*Calories Don't Count*

*Drink, Eat and Get Thin*

*Martinis and Whipped Cream Diet*

*The Doctor's Quick Weight Loss Diet*

*Dr. Atkin's Diet Revolution*

*The High Calorie Way To Stay Thin Forever*

*Fasting: The Ultimate Diet*

*Fit for Life*

*The Rotation Diet*

*Dr. Berger's Immune Power Diet*

*The T-Factor Diet*

These titles and advertising slogans reveal many things, if you really think about them. They attempt to present "facts" about losing weight. Unfortunately, the "facts" are usually lies. There are three major lies presented over and over again to the American public:

Lie 1: Losing weight is a good, appropriate, moral thing to do.

Lie 2: Losing weight is simple. It's easy. Anyone can do it.

Lie 3: If you do not lose weight quickly, easily, and keep it off forever, you are either bad or dumb.

Let's consider each of these lies and examine some alternative ways of thinking about them.

## Lie 1: Losing Weight Is a Good, Appropriate, Moral Thing To Do

The weight control industry tells you that you *really must* lose weight if you're overweight or if you even think you're overweight. This is considered especially true if you are a woman. Certainly the advertisers for the multibillion-dollar weight control industry do not come right out and say this. They say, instead, a variety of other things about the healthiness of being thin and active. They also show a sad, pathetic existence for people who are overweight. The frequency of advertisements and number of products for weight control also make this point. In other words, why would there be so many products, books, and programs about weight loss if it weren't an incredibly important, moral thing to do?

The truth is that losing weight is not a moral requirement for anybody! Do you see the same moral outrage presented to the public about the use of seatbelts? Why not? After all, a majority of Americans still do not use seatbelts, and, as a result, many Americans die in automobile accidents every year. What about the use of motorcycle helmets? This is another clear case of a very dangerous problem in America that is almost never discussed in the media. Consider a subject closer in many ways to weight control—exercise. The benefits and importance of exercise do not receive the same degree of attention as the importance of losing weight. Part of the explanation for these discrepancies is financial. Weight control is big business. Actually, it's very big business. From the time of early adolescence to old age, most women in the United States try to lose weight, often over and over again. Many millions of boys and men also diet and attempt to lose weight throughout their lives. These tens of millions of potential consumers of weight control ideas and products fuel an industry that will be worth $50 billion a year by the year 2000. This makes weight control very important to many, many people. Both weight controllers and those who sell to weight controllers have joined forces to make losing weight an incredibly important thing to do.

The degree to which losing weight is important depends on values. To people who lived at the turn of the century, or even in the 1950s, weight control and thinness were less important goals. Despite the increased emphasis on physical fitness today, thinness remains the ideal—especially for women. The implications for physical health of maintaining a low body weight are complicated. Excess weight does increase health risks. Yet to what degree is your health the major reason that you're reading this book? Almost all of the hundreds of people I have known who were making a serious effort to lose weight told me that their appearance was far more important than their health. Most people want to lose weight to change the way they look. They may recognize that excess weight causes health problems, but that does not drive them to spend $50 billion. They want to look good. Our society makes it clear that everybody *should* look good at all times. This creates a very powerful incentive for overweight people to change, to conform to the ideal, or to die trying.

The enormous cultural pressure toward thinness, especially for women, will not change easily. Certainly this book will not change that pressure. But you can make a conscious decision about your own willingness to accept that cultural standard. Remember, this cultural obsession with thinness is arbitrary. It changes over the decades. It does not have your best interests at heart. You may decide to work to become thinner to feel more accepted in our society. That is your choice. For most people who have a weight problem, that choice also makes sense from a health perspective. It also makes sense to work toward becoming more physically fit. Very few Americans are currently as physically fit as they could be to maximize their health and well-being. The important thing to remember is that when you decide to lose weight, you are making an active, personal choice.

My experience has shown that people who attempt to lose weight because they believe that losing weight is the moral, the good, or the right thing to do usually fail. If, on the other hand, you make an active choice to control your weight because you have decided it is the right thing for you, then you're taking a step toward persistence. People tend to rebel against an authoritarian "order"; whereas when they do things because they've made very active choices and decisions, they can move forward toward change. Marcia's case history illustrates this point.

## Case History: Marcia's Choice

One of my clients, Marcia, broke her ankle in an automobile accident. Marcia had been a very active individual and was extremely upset by the disability created by this accident. She had difficulty walking for many months. She "turned to food." Marcia was approximately 75 pounds overweight when I first met her almost ten years ago. She described her desire to lose weight as something she "had to do because I'm so fat." This feeling of being forced to lose weight seemed culturally based and not something Marcia actively chose to do. She set an unrealistic goal for her weight loss. She wanted to weigh the same as when she graduated from high school (more than 25 years ago). When asked about this excessively high standard for success, Marcia had difficulty acknowledging that it was unreasonable.

Marcia lost approximately 50 pounds and has kept it off for most of the last ten years. Her weight only fluctuated by 10 or 20 pounds throughout this time. She became a committed exerciser (although she says "I will never say 'I like it.' If I could stop exercising tomorrow and maintain this weight, I would do it so fast it would make your head spin!"). Over the years, she gradually changed her position about what she "had to weigh." She became more accepting of the limitations of her lifestyle and the relative unimportance of weighing what she had in high school. Although to this day she would prefer losing another 20 to 30 pounds, she is no longer driven toward an unreasonable goal. She has accepted a different standard for herself. Marcia seems happier with this kind of acceptance. She has rejected society's arbitrary standards of thinness for women and selected a compromise. It allows her to look better, feel more accepted by others, and be physically healthier and stronger. Her standard does not fit with our culture's ideal, but it is something she can live with.

## Lie 2: Losing Weight Is Easy. It's Simple. Anyone Can Do it.

Not only does the weight control industry say that losing weight is easy; most weight controllers have told me the same thing. The version that I hear from hundreds of people is, "Losing weight is easy; keeping it off is hard." Although I have heard this hundreds of times, when I work with people over periods of weeks, months, and years, it seems that losing weight is very difficult indeed. There may be periods of time, often brief at that, during which the weight loss process seems relatively easy. But weight controllers almost always struggle with some aspect of the process.

Certainly the weight control industry wants you to believe that losing weight is easy. If you believe that their program, or book, or product makes losing weight easy, you would be more likely to spend ten dollars, twenty dollars, or hundreds of dollars on their products. The following exercise will help you understand more fully the true nature of the battle.

---

### Four Causes of Problems With Weight Control

Why do you have a weight problem? The following factors all have something to do with it:

a. **Food and exercise**. The kind of food you eat and how much you exercise affect your weight.

b. **Family and friends**. How your family and friends eat and exercise and how important they consider exercise to be affect your weight.

c. **Emotions**. Eating because you feel upset or unable to handle stress, or because of other problems, affects your weight.

d. **Biology**. Your body (for example, the rate at which you burn calories, the number of fat cells you have), and the fact that you seem to gain weight faster and easier than others who eat and exercise just like you, affects your weight.

Which of these factors is most important? Compare their importance by filling in the blanks in the following list.

The most important factor is ___.

The second most important factor is ___.

The third most important factor is ___.

The fourth most important factor is ___.

Research suggests that all of these factors are important. But most people think that factor (d) (Biology) is far less important than it actually is. Experts say factor (d) is the single most important factor. Do you?

My answers for the second, third, and fourth most important factors are (a) food and exercise; (c) emotions; and (b) family and friends, respectively. No one can lose weight successfully while eating foods that are high in fat and sugar or while remaining sedentary. Emotional upsets can lead to binge eating and poor concentration. Healthy eating and exercising by family and friends encourages weight controllers to do the same.

## Biological Barriers to Weight Control

I have asked thousands of people to complete a version of this exercise. Some of these people were students, others were educators, some were physicians, and many were lifetime weight controllers. They all realized the importance of most of the factors, but less than 5 percent realized that biological factors were absolutely critical to weight control. An overwhelming amount of scientific evidence supports this assertion. Perhaps you have heard or read about some of the following biological factors that make permanent weight control so difficult:

- Fat cell number

- Fat cell size

- Lipoprotein lipase (LPL)

- Hyperinsulimia

- Adaptive thermogenesis

- Thermic effects of food

- Set-point

- Genetics

Each of these biological factors play some role in making weight control very difficult. Excess weight is essentially a biological problem. That is, when people develop excess weight, at any point in their lives, their bodies become especially efficient and effective at maintaining higher than normal levels of fat. The biological forces noted above include forces that you are born with (genetics), forces that develop throughout your life (fat cell size and number), and forces that work to maintain high levels of body fat (for example, set-points, adaptive thermogenesis, and thermic effects of food).

A few details about the biology of excess weight may help illustrate the power of this force. Terryl Foch and Gerald McClearn wrote a chapter in Albert Stunkard's book, *Obesity*, in which they summarized some of the evidence showing the genetic factors that affect obesity. "Genetic fac-

tors" are inherited, and they contribute to the way people look or function. Research indicates that mice can be selected for breeding so that
fatter mice mate with other fatter mice and leaner mice with other leaner
mice. This selective breeding program can produce mice pups from the
fatter matings with twice as much fat as the pups from the leaner matings.
It takes 15 to 25 matings (generations) to produce these different strains
of mice. This research shows the tremendous degree to which inheritance
or genetic makeup determines the tendency to develop excess fat.

Human parallels include research showing that children born to parents who are both obese are four times more likely to become obese than
children born to lean parents. Approximately 80 percent of children born
to obese parents become obese; while 40 percent of children born to one
obese and one lean parent, and 14 percent of children born to two lean
parents become obese.

Some recent research by Claude Bouchard also emphasizes the degree to which inheritance plays a role in developing excess weight. In
1990, Bouchard and his colleagues overfed 12 pairs of identical twins for
100 days. The twins lived in a closed hospital ward and consumed about
1000 calories per day above their normal intakes. Some pairs of twins
gained more that 25 pounds during those 100 days, whereas others who
were eating the same amounts gained less than 10 pounds. If one member
of a twin pair gained a lot of weight, the other member of the pair also
gained a lot of weight. In addition, the twins who gained more weight
tended to gain more of the weight as fat and less of it as lean body tissues
(such as muscles or organs). Other studies with twins who grow up in
separate households show similar trends. Twins who grow up in separate
households resemble each other in weight status much more than they
resemble the siblings with whom they grow up. These findings make it
clear that some of us are born to struggle with weight control, and others
are born to be lean.

Genetics do not determine everything about weight. Your family and
environment are also factors in weight control. For example, overweight
people are more likely to have overweight pets than leaner people. They
share absolutely no genetic material with their pets! Yet, something about
the way they live affects the obesity of their dogs and cats.

Beyond genetics, overweight people have many more fat cells and
other biological factors that encourage them to maintain higher weights.
Fat cells are like hungry baby sparrows clustered together in a nest. Both
sparrows and fat cells seem to open their "mouths" wider than their bodies in search of as much food as they can get. Once fat cells develop,
they never disappear. Overweight people can have four times as many
of these hungry "creatures" as their never-overweight, leaner peers. People can also develop more of these insatiable beasties at any point in their
lives. In fact, some research with animals shows that animals who "binge-
eat" (are fed large amounts of high-fat food) can permanently gain excess
fat cells within one week. These fat cells make use of the excess amounts

of insulin and the excess amounts of the cellular enzyme lipoprotein lipase (LPL) produced by overweight people. Insulin and LPL can keep fat cells as full as possible. In other words, overweight people have excess fat cells and other biological excesses (hormones and enzymes) that promote more efficient storage of fat than never-overweight people.

If you would like to know more details about these forces, you can find many readings listed in the Bibliography in the back of this book that discuss them (for example, see the book by Michael Perri and his colleagues, *Improving Long-Term Management of Obesity*, or *The Dieter's Dilemma*, by William Bennett and Joel Gurin). For now, it is not critical to review additional information about how these biological factors affect weight control. Rather, it is time to accept the fact that the biology of excess weight is a real and powerful force in the lives of every overweight individual. There is no escaping this reality. But you can learn to manage your biology effectively. *Biology is not destiny.*

## Biology Is Not Destiny

When I explained the biological forces against Joe, one of my clients, he became quite upset. Joe was stunned at the power of it all. He said, "I can't believe it! All of my life people, including doctors, told me I was normal. Now you're telling me that I'm biologically abnormal and that this biology is the main cause of my weight problem! This is too cruel to be true! Why did I have to live the last 20 years thinking I was so pathetic? It's not just me or my personality, right? I really have to live with something that's a physical force within me."

Joe's concerns are very legitimate. The biology of obesity takes no prisoners and takes no vacations. These biological forces are very real and powerful. When you think about it, this makes a lot of sense. Why would so many people have so much difficulty maintaining weight losses if biological forces did not oppose such weight losses? Losing weight produces many positive rewards. Relatively brief lapses of concentration (for example, binges and inconsistent exercising) are greeted very eagerly by your body's hungry fat cells. Most overweight people have many billions of fat cells more than people who never had weight problems. That's a lot of hungry sparrows to feed! These fat cells and other biological forces are always present and ready to take action.

The concerns expressed by Joe were heartfelt, but he came to appreciate the positive side of those concerns as well. That is, Joe had to first learn to accept the powerful role that biology plays in creating and maintaining weight problems. Once he accepted this, he could take some of the blame away from his own personality and self-esteem. He then recognized that persistence at weight control can help him manage this biological disorder. Like Joe, you do not have to overcome a "weak" and "pathetic" personality. You do not have to go from an abnormal state of gluttony to a normal state of controlled eating. Rather, you must change from a relatively normal state of functioning with an unfortunate biology to a super-normal state. Super-normal low-fat, low-calorie eating and frequent exercising are necessary to overcome the biology of obesity. This makes the challenge of weight control one of the most difficult challenges you can face.

## Lie 3: If You Do Not Lose Weight Quickly, Easily, and Keep It Off Forever, You Are Either Bad or Dumb

This is the biggest lie of all. It is the logical conclusion to the first two lies: Since losing weight is good and easy, you must be bad or dumb if you can't succeed. It's very personal. Overweight boys and girls experience this and suffer for it throughout their childhoods. Overweight adults also suffer needlessly because of this distorted view. It's the most unfair lie.

By now you know that it is best to consider losing weight as a personal choice. You *decide* if you want to live with the consequences of being overweight just as you decide whether or not to use seatbelts, whether or not to smoke, and whether or not to wear shabby clothes. If you decide to lose weight, nothing about it is easy. It takes super-normal skills of many kinds to persist effectively and lose weight. It can certainly be done, but it is never easy. If you are not successful at losing weight, you deserve sympathy, not damnation.

Consider how athletes are treated when they do not reach their goals. Did you know that only 3 percent of professional baseball players ever play, even for one minute, in the major leagues? Similar percentages of very talented and dedicated athletes ever make it to the higher echelons of their particular sports. Are athletes condemned for failing to be the best? No! They are praised for trying and congratulated for their dedication. This is exactly the approach that makes the most sense for all weight controllers. When athletes shape their bodies into a super-normal condition in order to achieve super-normal feats, they receive praise and support for the effort. When weight controllers shape their bodies into super-normal conditions via super-normal personal management skills, they deserve praise and support for the efforts. Essentially, *weight control is a major athletic challenge*. When weight controllers succeed, they deserve the same credit and admiration that we give to successful athletes. If they do not succeed, they deserve sympathy or at least acceptance. This is the best attitude to take toward yourself. If you make it and learn how to persist in order to control your weight, you deserve to feel very proud of accomplishing something remarkable. If you decide not to persist, you are neither bad nor dumb. You are simply human, and you are exercising your right to choose.

## The Three Truths

To summarize this section, let's take another look at the three lies and the truths that counteract them. Learning to reject these lies and replace them in your own thinking with these truths can help you pursue persistence at weight control. These truths can set you free to accept the realities of weight control and accept yourself.

**Lie 1:** You *really must* lose weight if you are overweight or if you even think you are overweight, especially if you are a woman. Losing weight is a good, appropriate, moral thing to do.

**Truth 1:** If you decide to lose weight, you are making a *choice*. You may choose to persist at weight control or you may choose not to lose weight. The decision is yours. This decision is not a moral or a religious one.

**Lie 2:** Losing weight is easy. It's simple. Anyone can do it.

**Truth 2:** Losing weight is very difficult. Losing weight requires super-normal eating, exercising, and personal management skills. Essentially, weight control is a major athletic challenge.

**Lie 3:** Since losing weight is good and easy, if you do not lose weight quickly, easily, and keep it off forever, you are either bad or dumb.

**Truth 3:** Since losing weight is very difficult, you deserve admiration and support for choosing to persist at this difficult biological challenge. If you succeed, you also deserve admiration. If you do not persist (and do not succeed at achieving and maintaining substantial weight loss), you deserve understanding and acceptance.

# All Personal Changes Are Challenging

Weight control may pose one of the greatest personal challenges that anyone could face, but all personal changes are challenging. As the illustration shows, everyone follows certain paths in their lives as a result of many very powerful influences. Your childhood, your genetic makeup, your early experiences, your relationships with significant people, your financial status, and many other factors move you toward walking down a certain road. Trying to get to a different road or pathway takes great effort and a little luck. Consider some of the following statistics about the manner in which people change:

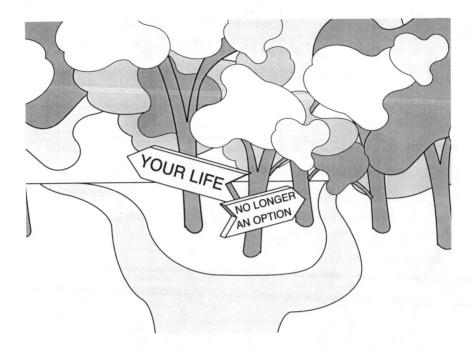

- **Prescriptions**. Approximately one-third of the 750 million new prescriptions written in a recent year in the United States and England were never filled. An additional 300 million of those prescriptions were not followed in the way they were written.

- **Adolescent cancer**. Approximately 50 percent of the medications prescribed to adolescents with cancer are not taken as directed.

- **Epilepsy**. Approximately 35 percent of the drug regimens prescribed for epilepsy are not followed.

- **Pediatric illness**. Parents fail to ensure that their children adhere to medication regimens approximately 50 percent of the time.

- **Behavior modification for children**. Approximately 50 percent of the parents involved with behavior modification programs for decreasing childhood problems discontinue the procedures against therapeutic advice.

- **Depression**. Approximately one-third of patients with manic-depressive disorders discontinue their medications against medical advice.

- **Schizophrenia**. Approximately 75 percent of schizophrenic patients discontinue treatment prematurely.

- **Chronic illnesses among the elderly**. A majority of elderly people who have chronic illnesses do not follow their prescribed and necessary medication regimens.

- **Kidney disease**. Approximately 70 percent of patients with kidney disease fail to follow dietary and fluid restrictions necessary for their comfort and health.

- **Seatbelts**. Approximately 65 percent of people fail to use seatbelts consistently.

- **High blood pressure**. Only 30 percent of people with high blood pressure follow the medical regimens that can save their lives.

- **Exercise**. Only 20 percent of adult Americans exercise at least twice a week for at least 30 minutes. The American College of Sports Medicine recommends that everyone should exercise at least four times per week.

- **Diabetes**. About 97 percent of diabetic patients adhere to all of the steps considered necessary for good control of this deadly disease.

These statistics startle some people. I've heard questions like, "How could people fail to take medications and follow other steps that are so critical to preserving their health and well-being?" In some ways, this perfectly reasonable question misses the point. The fact is that people usually struggle to maintain regimens of any kind that are different from what they are used to doing. Almost regardless of the consequences, people resist change mightily.

These statistics raise an important issue about weight control. Since people usually struggle to change their lifestyles, why are obese people blamed so harshly for problems that they encounter when trying to make huge changes in their lives? The answer comes from the way people think. People often develop biases about certain topics when they become emotionally involved in them. People become involved in weight control because it is emphasized so much in our culture. Also, they become involved because they see many people who gain and lose weight over and over again. Very few problems, if any, are as visible as weight problems. Many people decide that since many people regain the weight they lose, weight loss is impossible. "Since Mary, Jane, and Tim all regained the weight they lost, no one can do it," or so the thinking goes. This is distorted thinking. After all, people resist making changes in their lives. Why should weight control be any different? Weight control is *not* different. You can expect to have difficulty persisting with any major change that you attempt. Some people will not succeed. This does not mean that *you* cannot succeed. Persistence is challenging.

Weight controllers get an especially large dose of pessimism from others. The distortions in thinking about weight control come, in part, from blaming overweight people for their problems. Children as well as adults blame overweight individuals for their excess weight. If someone is an epileptic or diabetic, they are considered blameless and unfortunate; people do not understand that powerful biological forces make weight control very challenging. They see excess weight as a product of gluttony and personal inadequacy. Have you heard this gem? "If you are overweight, you must eat too much and you must be too lazy or too weak to change." Remember that persistence makes change possible. Athletes can become highly skilled; diabetics can control all aspects of their disease effectively; people with high blood pressure can control it; children can take their medications as prescribed; and overweight people can become healthier and slimmer. None of these things is easy, but all of them are possible—with commitment and persistence.

## Committing to Change

How committed are you to losing weight? Is it one of the top two or three priorities in your life right now? Or does it fall somewhere much farther down the list? Part of the answer to these questions comes from considering the advantages and disadvantages of attempting to lose weight. When you thoroughly analyze the possible advantages and disadvantages of a particular goal, you become more committed to that goal. This commitment leads to greater persistence.

### The Decision Balance Technique

The "Decision Balance Sheet" on the next page asks you to write out the positive and negative aspects of trying to reach your weight loss goal. First, write in a specific goal for the next year. For example, are you trying to lose 20, or 50, or 100 pounds during this next year? When writing out the goal, consider that it works best to state a goal that is difficult but achievable. It is extremely difficult for anybody to lose 100 pounds in one year, regardless of the methods used. For most people, realistic goals for weight loss include losing between one-quarter and one pound per week. After stating your goal, write out everything you can think of that would be good or positive about attempting to reach that goal. What effects on your life would reaching that goal have and what would you enjoy about those effects? After writing out the positive side of this decision, consider the negatives as well. Weight control takes time, effort, and money for everyone who seeks it. What are the specific costs to you of attempting to lose weight this year? Spend a few minutes writing out the positives and negatives of attempting to lose weight.

Jan completed her Decision Balance Sheet in an unusual way. She divided the positive and negative consequences of attempting to lose weight into several categories. You can see on the following pages that these categories include tangible or material gains and losses to herself and to others. They also include anticipations that are personal or social, not material.

# Decision Balance Sheet

Name:_____ Date:_____

Goal:_____

*Positive Aspects of Trying to Reach the Goal and About Reaching
the Goal*

1. _____
2. _____
3. _____
4. _____
5. _____
6. _____
7. _____
8. _____
9. _____
10. _____

*Negative Aspects of Trying to Reach the Goal and About Reaching
the Goal*

1. _____
2. _____
3. _____
4. _____
5. _____
6. _____
7. _____
8. _____
9. _____
10. _____

It might be helpful to you to examine Jan's list. After studying Jan's list, consider revising your own Decision Balance Sheet. It helps to include all the factors that might result from attempting to lose weight when making a decision as challenging as this one.

After considering your decision very carefully, determine how committed you are to losing weight. Do your positive anticipations clearly outweigh your negative anticipations? This analysis requires not just a simple count of positive versus negative anticipations, it requires you to study the importance of each item on your list. In Jan's case, improved job opportunities and improved abilities to be active were extremely important to her. As a 54-year-old woman who was more than 100 pounds overweight, her knees and back had become more than minor annoyances. These problems affected her ability to spend time with people who were important to her and to do many things that she wanted to do.

For example, Jan is a high school teacher who loves to travel. During her long summer vacations, she has not been able to travel in the last two years because of complications associated with her weight problem. Traveling was important to her husband and to herself. She very much wanted to change this limitation imposed by her weight. She wanted to reverse the aging process that had essentially become accelerated due to her weight problems.

She had become "old before her time." She was functioning as an 80-year-old instead of a 54-year-old. Jan's positive anticipations were far more significant to her than all of the negative anticipations. So, when Jan asked herself about her commitment to change, she realized that it was very strong. When you examine your own commitment, consider the degree to which the positive anticipations are more important to you than the negative ones.

---

### Jan's Decision Balance Sheet
### Goal: Lose 50 pounds in one year
#### Tangible Gains/Losses to Self

*Positive Anticipations*
1. Improve ability to walk around, shop, bike.
2. Improve tennis game.
3. Increase contact with others.
4. Improve health in long run (live longer!).
5. Increase job opportunities.
6. Be able to buy more stylish clothes.
7. Be able to borrow others' clothes.
8. Go to the beach more.
9. Get presents other than stationery (like clothes!).
10. Spend less money on fad diets, specialized diet foods.

## Jan's Decision Balance Sheet (continued)
### Tangible Gains/Losses to Self

*Negative Anticipations*

1. Takes lots of time to count calories, monitor food.
2. Costs money for group sessions, exercise classes.
3. Exercising may cause injuries.
4. Takes time to keep records and do exercise.
5. Costs money for new clothes.
6. _____
7. _____
8. _____
9. _____
10. _____

### Tangible Gains/Losses to Others

*Positive Anticipations*

1. Increase socializing (helping others, being a friend).
2. More energy for family.
3. More willing to do active things with family.
4. More expertise available for family in nutrition, exercise, self-control.
5. More expertise available for friends.
6. I may live longer, so I can help my family longer.
7. More healthful foods and lifestyle modeled by me for family.
8. _____
9. _____
10. _____

*Negative Anticipations*

1. I may burden others with need for support.
2. Others in family will have to do more cooking.
3. I'll be busier—with exercising and group sessions—so less time for others.
4. There will be fewer "treats" available in the house.
5. There will be less money available for others.
6. _____
7. _____
8. _____
9. _____
10. _____

## Jan's Decision Balance Sheet (continued)
### Self-Approval/Disapproval

*Positive Anticipations*
1. Feel proud.
2. Feel more self-confident.
3. Feel sense of mastery.
4. Feel in control of my body.
5. Understand my body and myself better.
6. _____
7. _____
8. _____
9. _____
10. _____

*Negative Anticipations*
1. Feel too "obsessed."
2. Feel restricted.
3. Become less joyful and spontaneous.
4. Will have bought into cultural pressures to be thin.
5. Feel too much like a "health nut."
6. _____
7. _____
8. _____
9. _____
10. _____

### Social Approval/Disapproval

*Positive Anticipations*
1. Friends will congratulate me.
2. Relatives will recognize my strengths.
3. People will see me as a person first, and not just as a "fat person."
4. Kids won't laugh at me anymore.
5. Spouse will find me more attractive.
6. Increased attractiveness to others.
7. Friends will like my less depressed, happier disposition.
8. _____
9. _____
10. _____

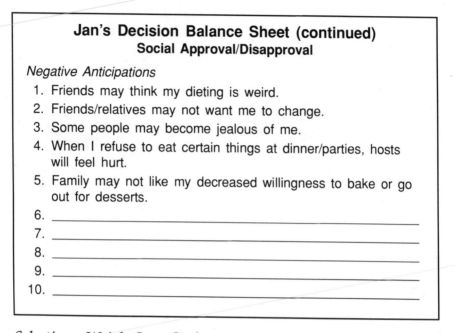

**Jan's Decision Balance Sheet (continued)**
**Social Approval/Disapproval**

*Negative Anticipations*

1. Friends may think my dieting is weird.
2. Friends/relatives may not want me to change.
3. Some people may become jealous of me.
4. When I refuse to eat certain things at dinner/parties, hosts will feel hurt.
5. Family may not like my decreased willingness to bake or go out for desserts.
6. _____
7. _____
8. _____
9. _____
10. _____

## Selecting a Weight Loss Goal

Jan selected a weight loss goal of 50 pounds over the course of the year. She actually needed to lose more weight than that (approximately 80 pounds). Selecting an appropriate goal for weight loss presents its own unique challenges. A wide variety of tables and recommendations exist that could lead to dramatically different goals. I recommend using Table I (shown on page 26) when selecting your goal. This table, from the U.S. Departments of Agriculture and Health and Human Services, presents a wide range of desirable weights for people in two different age categories: 19 to 34 years old and 35 years and older. The weights listed are based on heights measured without shoes and weights measured without clothes.

You'll notice that this is perhaps the first "suggested weights" table you have ever seen that does not distinguish between men and women. This table is based strictly on research showing which weights associated with which heights predicted good health in the long run. It turned out that sex did *not* predict health in this research. That is, for a 5-foot-4-inch woman, you will note that the weight range of 111 to 146 pounds is listed. Any weight within that range is associated with relatively low risks of health problems in the long run. Of course, the lower weight ranges are the ones that generally apply to women (who generally have less muscle and smaller and less dense bones). A reasonable goal for a 5-foot-4-inch woman is a weight somewhere near the lower side of the range listed for her height and age. If this woman were 42 years old, for example, she might select 130 pounds as a reasonable goal. This goal is higher than the cultural ideal, but it is associated with good health and may be more attainable than the lower and more questionable weights that many people would select on their own.

This table also shows that as people get older, higher weights are more typical and perfectly acceptable. As people age, their metabolic rates slow down, and they tend to increase fat and lose some muscle and bone. This results in higher overall weights. If you remain physically fit, you can actually benefit from having a few extra pounds on your body. Having more rather than too few pounds aids recovery from surgeries, heart attacks, and other traumas. Since older people tend to experience more of such traumas, somewhat higher weights produce better health overall for those individuals.

Another aspect of weight loss goals is illustrated in the following graph. Note that the "average person" tends to gain a pound or so per year. Some research suggests that many overweight people gain several pounds per year. When you select a weight loss goal and plan to get there and stay there for years, you are bucking this trend. The "you" line on the graph shows that your goal is ambitious. Overweight people tend to gain weight over time—that's normal. It will take consistent effort to become super-normal—to become a successful weight controller.

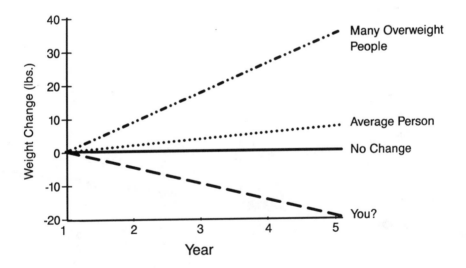

## Reaffirming Your Commitment

Your Decision Balance Sheet can remain an active part of the weight control process. Review these lists over and over again as you attempt to lose weight. They serve as reminders of what really matters to you when the going gets rough. And the going always gets rough as you develop and refine your persistence at weight control. Everyone suffers

## Table I
## Suggested Weights for Adults

| Height | Weight in pounds | |
|---|---|---|
| | 19 to 34 years | 35 years and over |
| 5'0" | 97-128 | 108-138 |
| 5'1" | 101-132 | 111-143 |
| 5'2" | 104-137 | 115-148 |
| 5'3" | 107-141 | 119-152 |
| 5'4" | 111-146 | 122-157 |
| 5'5" | 114-150 | 126-162 |
| 5'6" | 118-155 | 130-167 |
| 5'7" | 121-160 | 134-172 |
| 5'8" | 125-164 | 138-178 |
| 5'9" | 129-169 | 142-183 |
| 5'10" | 132-174 | 146-188 |
| 5'11" | 136-179 | 151-194 |
| 6'0" | 140-184 | 155-199 |
| 6'1" | 144-489 | 159-205 |
| 6'2" | 148-195 | 164-210 |
| 6'3" | 152-200 | 168-216 |
| 6'4" | 156-205 | 173-222 |
| 6'5" | 160-211 | 177-228 |
| 6'6" | 164-216 | 182-234 |

setbacks. Those who succeed find ways of revitalizing their commitments, and thereby persisting. If you remember this, and continually refer to your Decision Balance Sheet, you can revitalize your own efforts when you want to intensify your commitment.

Some people cut out pictures from magazines to keep their focus strong. For example, Jan cut out pictures of Spain and Israel from travel magazines. She kept these on her refrigerator and in her office. They were gentle reminders about what she was trying to accomplish. She also concentrated on the movement of people around her. She noticed how easy it was for them to simply get up and go when they wanted to. This type of concentration had escaped her as she was gaining more weight and becoming more and more immobilized. Now she could look at people's movements and use it as an inspiration for her own commitment to persistence.

Jan used another technique that helps improve commitment. She wrote several key words, like the ones shown here, on the back of a business card and placed the card in her wallet.

Walking

Self-confidence

Mastery

Person first

Clothes

Health

Energy

Looks

Every time she took money out of her wallet, she also took a few seconds to review the card. Each of the eight points on the card meant something important to her. She spent a few seconds reflecting on the importance of weight control in her life by reviewing these points. For example, she affirmed how much she wanted others to consider her a "person first" instead of a "fat person first." Jan also wanted to feel more confident, develop mastery over this problem that had plagued her for a lifetime, and wear more interesting and attractive clothes. It only takes a few seconds to review these important goals. Persistence at weight control comes from many small efforts like this one.

Jan could have listed one, two, four, or ten points on her card. In fact, she changed cards many times over the years. One time she just wrote "PERSIST." Jan kept changing her "reminder cards" to keep herself interested in this approach. Why not try this technique yourself? By continually reminding yourself of the benefits that you may realize through improved weight control, you will make a stronger, clearer commitment.

## And So the Battle Begins (Again)

You may choose to persist at weight control or you may choose not to persist. The decision always remains yours. This decision is not a moral or a religious one. It is a personal choice. When choosing to lose weight you are choosing to develop super-normal eating, exercising, and personal management skills. These qualities are necessary to overcome the tenacious and resistant biology associated with excess weight. You can tame your biology. Biology is not destiny. Just as athletes overcome their bodies' resistance to demanding training and practice regimens, you can overcome your body's resistance to a lower weight. Losing weight is possible, but it is never easy. If you succeed at this challenging task, you deserve admiration. If you do not persist (and do not succeed at achieving and maintaining substantial weight loss), you deserve understanding and acceptance.

Weight control does not differ from any other efforts at personal change. Humans resist change. They spend their whole lives behaving and thinking and living in a certain way. Making major shifts in behavior requires very consistent and very persistent effort. The demands of almost any difficult personal challenge decrease when you understand the nature of the goal. This understanding includes identifying why you want to achieve it. The Decision Balance Sheet is a means of clarifying the positive and negative aspects of attempting to lose weight. When you review on a regular basis the specific reasons for making this difficult change in your life, you increase your commitment. It is very helpful to read that list every day. You can also modify your list on a regular basis. Using this technique can improve your commitment to persistence at weight control.

Rest assured that if any miracle cures are developed, you will hear about them. The media, your physicians, and other health care professionals would want you to know about such a wonderful thing. Meanwhile, you will benefit most from remaining committed to approaches that have scientific research behind them. These approaches offer no miracles. There is one exception to this: When you persist in the face of a very challenging task, you create your own miracle.

## Key Principles

- The multibillion-dollar weight control industry emphasizes (over and over again): You can lose weight easily and quickly! This is a grave exaggeration and oversimplification of the weight control process.

- There are three major lies promoted by the weight control industry: (1) you *really must* lose weight if you are overweight or if you even think you're overweight. Losing weight is always a good thing to do; (2) losing weight is easy; (3) since losing weight is good and easy, if you do not lose weight, you are either bad or dumb.

- Losing weight is a personal choice; losing weight is very difficult; if you decide to lose weight, you deserve admiration and support; if you decide not to persist, you deserve understanding acceptance.

- People usually struggle to make major changes in their lives, regardless of the consequences of not making them.

- You can improve your commitment to weight control by writing out the advantages and disadvantages of pursuing this goal.

# Epilogue

## Blind Resistance to Change

In their book *Facilitating Treatment Adherence*, Donald Meichenbaum and Dennis Turk describe a remarkable example of how people resist change despite sometimes dire consequences. They describe a study by Patricia Vincent on the serious, but very treatable, eye disease—glaucoma. Patients who were diagnosed with glaucoma were told that "they must use eye drops three times per day or *they would go blind*." Vincent reported that only 42 percent of these patients used the eye drops frequently enough to avoid permanent damage to their vision. Only 28 percent of the people who had not adhered adequately to the regimen improved their use of the eye drops even after they reached the point of becoming legally blind in one eye!

# 3

# The Stages of Change

"I think I can. I think I can. I think I can. . . . *I can!*"

versus

"I think I can't. I think I can't. I think I can't. . . . *I can't!*"

## Great (and Not so Great) Expectations

If people expect to succeed, they often do; if they expect to fail, they rarely succeed. These assertions are surprisingly accurate. Psychologists have studied the power of positive thinking for more than 60 years. Positive thinking alone cannot get you to walk an hour a day or order fruit instead of cheesecake. But positive thinking—believing in the possibility of positive change—works much better than pessimism. The following examples illustrate the wide range of situations in which expectations can affect outcomes. The first is from *Changing Expectations: A Key to Effective Psychotherapy,* by Irving Kirsch.

### Mind Over Taco

I always liked Mexican food, but I didn't like hot spicy food; in fact, I found the experience painful. Even a radish made me feel uncomfortable. I coped with this dilemma by frequenting Tex-Mex restaurants only in the gringo neighborhoods of Los Angeles, ordering just the safe foods—burritos, tostadas, cheese enchiladas, and frijoles. The hot sauce sat safely at the end of the table, untouched.

"Have you ever been to El Tippiac?" Mike Wapner asked, following one of our rambling afternoon excursions down the twisting lanes of theoretical psychology.

I shook my head.

"You've got to try it," he said exuberantly. "They make the best tacos in the world."

This was too promising to pass up. We collected Nancy, Michael's wife and colleague, and the three of us went to El Tippiac, where we ordered guacamole tacos. Mike and Nancy began eating theirs with gusto, and I bit into mine with eager anticipation.

When you take your first bite of a hot dish, there is a short period of time during which you can taste the flavor of the food, before it is eclipsed by the fiery sensation of the spice. During that brief delay, the delicious flavor of the guacamole taco came through. But then came the pain—excruciating pain! A familiar searing sensation spread through my mouth, and my eyes began to water.

Normally at that point, I would swallow the offending substance as quickly as possible and grope for a glass of water. But that afternoon, I did not. A sudden insight had occurred to me. Recalling the marvelous flavor that the pain had obscured, and seeing the expressions of pleasure on the faces of my friends, I thought: "Why am I experiencing pain while they are experiencing pleasure? The tacos are the same, and there is nothing physically different between them and me. We have the same kinds of taste buds, the same type of pain receptors. It's not fair! I too should be able to enjoy a guacamole taco."

Thinking back to that experience, I realize that my conclusions were not entirely sound. Perhaps there is a physiological difference between people who enjoy spicy foods and those who find them painful. Yet at the time, I had no doubts. I was certain that the difference was not physiological, and I decided to experience exactly what they were experiencing.

So I did not swallow as quickly, nor did I reach for a glass of water. Instead, I chewed slowly. I rolled the food around in my mouth. I savored it.

And then a strange thing happened. The taco still tasted spicy, but the spiciness was no longer painful. It began to feel pleasant, and finally, wonderful.

From that day on, my experience of spicy food has been different; it is no longer painful. When it is good and spicy, it is spicy and good.

The next three examples are based on studies involving arm wrestling by L. Nelson and M. Furst in 1972, skin irritations by Y. Ikemi and

S. Nakagawa in 1962, and dental procedures by S. Dworkin and his co-workers in 1984.

## Mind Over Muscle

Twenty-four men were tested for arm strength. These men were also asked to rate their strength compared to each of the other 23 men in the study. Subjects were then paired and asked to arm wrestle each other. The researchers arranged the pairs so that one man was clearly stronger than the other. However, both men believed that the stronger man was actually weaker. Ten of the 12 contests (83 percent) were won by the man who tested weaker! The experiment was set up so that both opponents expected these weaker men to win. These results suggest that expectations can overcome physical strength.

## Mind Over Poison Ivy

Thirteen boys were touched on their left arms with leaves that looked like poison ivy. These leaves were harmless, but the boys were told the leaves sometimes caused irritations to the skin. They were touched on their right arms with leaves that they believed were harmless. Actually, these leaves were from a plant that creates a skin rash similar to poison ivy (from a lacquer or wax tree). So, "reality" suggests that none of the boys should have developed any skin reactions on their left arms. All of them should have developed reactions on their right arms. These "shoulds" are based on the actual qualities of the leaves themselves. Amazingly, all 13 boys developed a skin reaction to the harmless leaves (on their left arms). Only two reacted to the leaves from the wax tree on their right arms. Here again, expectations overcame "reality."

## Mind Over Pain

Dentists often use nitrous oxide (laughing gas) to alter consciousness and reduce pain. Several researchers told one group of dental patients that the nitrous oxide "lowers the brain's level of consciousness about anxiety and pain, making people feel good ... your toes, maybe your hands, may begin tingling, and a kind of warm glow may come over you, a feeling of relaxation of muscle tension. These signs from your body, which compare with drinking a glass of wine or even smoking marijuana, indicate that the nitrous oxide has reached physiologically active levels. The drug is now working." This group reported relatively low amounts of pain and unpleasant physical sensations after receiving nitrous oxide. The second group was told that the altered state of consciousness produced by nitrous oxide can increase certain sensations, creating "a kind of exclusive awareness of what's going on in the body." This group reported significantly more pain than the first group. In other words, laughing gas alone affects sensations. If people believe those sensations decrease pain, they feel less pain during dental procedures. When the people believe that those sensations increase their awareness, they report greater amounts of pain during the dental procedures. Expectations clearly influence perceptions of pain.

These examples of the power of expectations apply directly to weight control. What do you expect right now from your efforts at weight control? Are your expectations more like Jane's or Barbara's?

Jane: "I really can't imagine living my life on a diet. I think people have to experiment with their eating. I just need to eat burgers and french fries sometimes. I also can't imagine exercising everyday or even almost every day. What if I just don't feel like exercising sometimes? I'm not sure if I'm ready to live my life like a nun."

Barbara: "I would love to learn how to actually enjoy exercising. I have never exercised consistently. I think I can learn to focus on exercising and find a way to make exercising a part of my life. There are times when I actually seem to prefer eating in the right way, as well. I am hoping and expecting that I can make low-fat eating a part of my daily routine. I don't want to keep fighting it anymore."

If your expectations are more like Jane's than Barbara's, you have a lot of work to do. Jane expects to struggle and seems to resent the process. Barbara expects to change and seems to look forward to the process. Perhaps it would make sense for Jane to talk with people who have become effective weight controllers. She would find that many of them take pride in their abilities to control their eating and exercising. Successful weight controllers also feel good after exercising. Even people who have not overcome weight problems learn to enjoy the way it feels to exercise and the health benefits that exercising brings. If Jane talks with committed exercisers and successful weight controllers, she may find it possible to achieve success. If she reads about these topics, that may help as well. However, if she cannot believe that she is capable of making the difficult changes required to succeed, she has very little chance of achieving substantial weight loss. Barbara, on the other hand, can envision her life as a successful weight controller. She expects to succeed. This positive expectation can help.

## Expectations for Successful Weight Control

What would happen if you expected to lose 100 pounds in one year and you "only" lost 30? What would happen if you expected to remain optimistic and positive when pursuing effective weight control, and you found yourself becoming annoyed and frustrated with the process? These are examples of positive expectations about a task as difficult as persistence at weight control. But it helps even more to tailor these positive expectations to the reality of the process. The road to successful weight control is bumpy. It helps to understand and anticipate the nature of the bumps and how to cope with them. Developing a good understanding of what to expect can improve commitment and persistence.

My colleagues and I have noticed that weight controllers tend to experience certain phases or stages along the way to successful persistence. The experiences of hundreds of weight controllers has contributed to the development of this model of the stages of change in successful weight control. This model can help you refine your understanding about what to expect during the difficult journey ahead.

The illustration on the next page shows the three primary and three secondary stages of the model. Each stage consists of characteristic, or typical, behaviors, thoughts, and feelings. That is, people in each stage tend to act and think in similar ways. By no means do all people experience all six stages. However, you may find it useful to consider the nature of each stage. You can decide whether these stages describe your previous experiences when pursuing weight control.

The primary stages seem to be experienced by most people during the first two years of committed effort at weight control. The secondary stages seem to affect less than 20 percent of those who seek long-term weight control. Let's review the definitions of each of the primary stages first and then consider the secondary stages.

## Primary Stages of Weight Control

### Honeymoon

**Thoughts and feelings**  Weight controllers in this stage often express delight and a sense of genuine satisfaction. They seem relieved and eager to take control of this difficult problem.

**Behaviors**  Honeymooners consistently attend weight control sessions (if they're participating in a formal program). They also carefully observe themselves by keeping records of their eating and exercising. They read about weight control and exercise. Honeymooners also talk with other people about health, weight control, and related topics.

**Example**  Lisa was a 35-year-old nurse who was married and had two young children when I first met her. She had a busy and very fulfilling life. Unfortunately, she broke her leg in several places one day in a serious car accident. That day led to a great deal of pain and a long recovery. Before the accident, Lisa's weight was never what she wanted it to be. It was just on the high side of the normal range. For six months

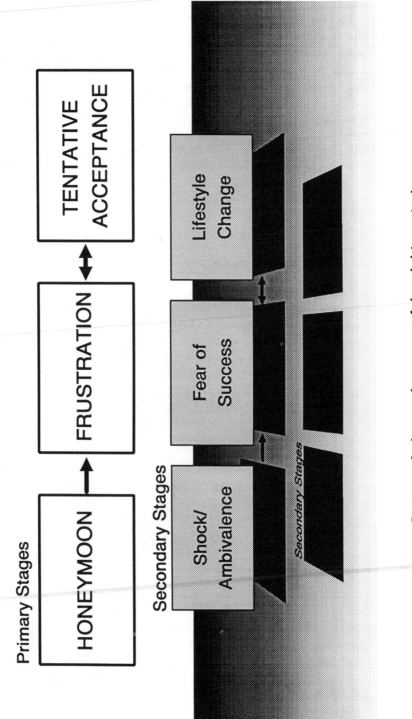

Stages of change in successful weight control

after the accident she struggled to rehabilitate her leg. She went to physical therapy three times a week. She had to cope with the boredom that comes with restricted mobility on the weekends. Lisa gained 50 pounds during that six-month recovery. She described much of her eating as "something to soothe me. It helped me feel less bored and happier—at least for a little while." Eating ice cream and cookies became a means of coping. She realized that her feelings of frustration and boredom led to problematic eating. Unfortunately, she did not find more adaptive methods of coping.

Lisa began participating in a therapy group that I conducted soon after her leg had healed completely. She was annoyed, angry, depressed, and eager to change. She grasped onto the ideas and principles that were discussed in the group. She kept meticulous records of what she ate and when she exercised. Lisa was pursuing persistence at weight control. She was "going for it!" She seemed very committed, dedicated, and happy to have a chance to tame this difficult problem.

Lisa's monitoring of her eating and exercising remained meticulous and complete for about 12 months. She did not resent the effort that it required for her to achieve a 60-pound weight loss during that year. She showed remarkable enthusiasm and concentration. Weight loss became a focal point for her. Lisa's attitude and efforts also helped encourage and inspire the rest of the group members.

### Frustration

**Thoughts and feelings** In this stage, people often think about going back to their old ways of eating and exercising. They long for the old days. After all, the old ways are easier and take much less time and energy. People in the Frustration stage resent the effort required for successful weight control. They compare themselves to people who are not overweight and people who have never been overweight. This is a "why me?" stage. "Why do I have to work at this all the time?" "Why can't I take a break from the effort every once in a while?" "Why doesn't my spouse have to suffer with this biology?" In this stage, weight controllers battle life's basic unfairness.

**Behaviors** Weight controllers in this stage become less careful about their eating and exercising. They do not monitor their eating and exercising as well as they did in the Honeymoon stage. If they are attending a formal program, they may have more difficulties getting to their meetings and getting there on time. The expression "hanging in there" (sometimes, just barely) describes this well.

**Example** Lisa, the same woman in the Honeymoon example, eventually reached the Frustration stage. About a year or so after a great deal of hard work, dedication, and effectiveness at weight control, she began struggling. During this stage, she talked about resenting how easy it was for her husband to "eat whatever he wants." Her rate of weight loss slowed, and it became more difficult for her to keep accurate records of her eating and exercising. She refused to give up, but her feelings changed from eagerness to frustration. "Why me?" was a consistent theme in Lisa's comments in the group. She could not understand or accept her rate of weight loss either. The year before, if she didn't lose weight during one particular week, she would say, "No problem. It'll happen. I'm on track." In this stage, she said, "I can't believe this! I'm eating practically nothing and look what happens! Nothing!"

### Tentative Acceptance

**Thoughts and feelings** This is a stage in which people settle in for the long haul. They experience *a peaceful sense of resolve* about weight control. They feel comfortable, with a clear direction for handling their challenging biologies. They also refine their knowledge of nutrition in this stage. Their understanding of the factors that affect weight control becomes clearer, as well. They still struggle with their focusing or commitment, however. This happens quite often when they go on vacations or when their schedules are disrupted by illness or travel.

**Behaviors** When weight controllers reach the Tentative Acceptance stage, they have developed very consistent patterns of exercise. They view exercise as either enjoyable or at least acceptable. They no longer see it as drudgery, but as something that can help them. So they maintain more positive and effective attitudes toward it.

In this stage, weight controllers consistently monitor their food and exercise. They also assert themselves effectively in restaurants and other social situations regarding food. For example, weight controllers in this stage would not accept a meal ordered "grilled, as dry as possible" if it were served swimming in butter. They would ask their server to have the fish or chicken reprepared. Weight controllers in the Tentative Acceptance stage do not battle themselves anymore about ordering low-fat, low-calorie meals. They do not feel deprived and frustrated when they ask for their food to be prepared in a healthful way. They feel taken care of and happier when they can get food prepared the way they now "prefer." I put the word "prefer" in quotes very deliberately. Can you really prefer baked potatoes to french fries? Fresh berries to chocolate mousse? Cheeseless pizza to sausage or pepperoni (and cheese, of course) pizza? Most people in this stage might say, "No way! I'll eat the healthier alternatives, but no one can convince me that low fat tastes better than high fat. Be real!"

Weight controllers in this stage still struggle with certain situations and still experience eating and exercising lapses (even binges occasionally). Just as disruptions in routines (vacations, travel) alter commitment or focus, these disruptions change behaviors too. Travel and vacations change routines and rules. Snacking during the day, for example, may not occur during a typical work week. During vacations, on the other hand, the opportunities to snack increase, and the "I deserve it" rationales reemerge.

**Example**  Lisa, the woman discussed in the previous stages, came out of the Frustration stage and went into the Tentative Acceptance stage. She began to realize that her frustration was getting her nowhere. Sure, her biology was much more difficult to manage than her husband's and other more fortunate people around her. Who said life was fair? She saw the challenge before her as something that she could accomplish. She realized that she had maintained a substantial weight loss. Even if she never lost another pound, she noted, at least she was not gaining weight anymore. She can now fit into many more of her clothes and feels better about herself. Lisa's feelings shifted from frustration and anger to a calmer, more peaceful state. She still had a lot of trouble with vacations and other major disruptions in her routines. During these times she developed a "vacation mentality." This "give myself a break" attitude led to more problematic eating. She recovered from these lapses very effectively, however. She restarted her monitoring of eating and exercising as soon as she got home. She reinforced her own refusal to give up. She could even laugh about her vacation mentality. She realized that her fat cells take no vacations. They remain ever-eager to pounce on those extra calories. They love her vacations!

### Living Within the Primary Stages

The three primary stages of weight control help describe the nature of persistence at weight control over long periods of time. Sometimes things go well, and other times the struggle becomes hard to tolerate. After a while, most persistent weight controllers get to "Tentative Acceptance or beyond. The doubleheaded arrow in the picture of the stages of change demonstrates that people sometimes move back and forth between the Frustration and the Tentative Acceptance stages. Sometimes they are very accepting of the problem and challenges of weight control; at other times, they become frustrated and annoyed at the whole thing. If they've achieved genuine persistence, they find a way to "hang in there" during Frustration and spend more and more time in Tentative Acceptance. You can expect to experience most of these primary stages in your future as a persistent weight controller.

## Secondary Stages of Weight Control

### Shock and Ambivalence

**Thoughts and feelings**  Sometimes weight controllers react with surprise and even anger about the nature of the battle that they must face with their own bodies. Persistence is not easy. Generally, in American culture, people are used to getting what they want when they want it.

Weight control simply does not work that way. In this secondary stage, weight controllers sometimes become particularly skeptical about the value of working so hard for so long. They seem very disappointed and annoyed. "There must be an easier way of doing this" describes the key statement in the Shock and Ambivalence stage.

**Behaviors**  Weight controllers may jump from one approach to another during this stage. They may try one commercial program or another, or join one health club or another, or try a professional program and then drop out of it. The quest for "the quick fix" characterizes this stage.

**Example**  Ed was a 48-year-old executive in a major corporation when I first met him. He was approximately 80 pounds overweight and had high blood pressure. Ed was married and he had two boys whom he loved dearly. He became increasingly concerned about the problems associated with his weight. His back frequently "went out," and his doctor was very concerned about his blood pressure. Ed realized that weight loss was critical to his happiness and vitality.

Ed participated in a group that I conducted. At first, he seemed enthusiastic and attempted to follow the guidelines in the program. He monitored his food intake and his exercise. He attempted to solve the problems that interfered with eating low-calorie foods and the problems associated with too little activity in his everyday life. After a few weeks of this rather positive "honeymoon," Ed began complaining. "Why can't I lose weight faster?" he would say. Even though Ed was losing approximately one pound per week, he would not accept that rate of weight loss. He reported losing several pounds a week on previous crash diets. His monitoring became more sporadic, and he started missing some group sessions. When he did come to the group, he had numerous excuses and continued to complain about the quality of the program. He eventually discontinued participation in the group. I attempted to reach him several times over the ensuing months. However, Ed did not return my phone calls nor did he respond to the letter I sent him.

Two years after discontinuing his work in the group, Ed gave me a call. His efforts were not successful and he was now 100 pounds overweight. His knees consistently bothered him and his hypertension was barely under control, even with medication. Ed scheduled an appointment to get back to the hard work of persisting at weight control. Unfortunately, he did not show up for his appointment and did not call again at any time during the next two years.

Ed's case illustrates the many challenges of persistence. Staying with the effort required by weight control does not fit comfortably in many people's lives. When people are used to getting things that they want quickly, they have to work very hard to tolerate the frustrations that are a natural part of effective weight control. It is sad when someone like Ed does not succeed. But remember, many athletes do not fulfill their potentials either. These individuals can find other sources of satisfaction in their lives. Most of the wonderfully gifted athletes in this country never get professional contracts, and those who do, often do not stay at the top of their games for very long. It is not an immoral or horrible thing to fail to persist at sports or weight control. It takes a lot of tolerance for frustration and often help from others to persist. Stay with it and you will be rewarded for the effort. If you do not persist, you have committed no sins. You can find ways of staying happy without this persistence.

### Fear of Success

**Thoughts and feelings**  Occasionally—actually very rarely—weight controllers worry about succeeding. They might worry about becoming too small or too sexy. Most people would love to become "too small" or "too sexy." For people in the Fear of Success stage, however, the thought of these changes produces anxiety and worry. Compliments from others about weight losses or changed appearances can trigger anxiety in some people.

**Behaviors**  Sometimes people in this stage sabotage their own efforts. They might eat with people who usually eat high-fat foods. They might begin cooking and baking too much. They might put themselves in situations that produce too much eating and not enough exercising. Their monitoring of eating and exercising behaviors may slip and they may begin to gain weight. They often eat in binges.

**Example**  One of my clients, George, once told me, "If I keep losing weight, I'll get too small. I'm used to being a big guy and a powerful force in meetings and discussions. I don't like the idea of being smaller and less noticeable. I'm just not comfortable with the idea of fitting in better."

Jane expressed a related concern: "I'm not used to men looking at me in a sexual way. Men are now approaching me differently and looking at me differently. I don't like it. I really don't know how to handle this."

These concerns make sense. George was used to being big and noticeable, and he enjoyed certain aspects of his size. Jane, on the other hand, was used to nonsexual relationships with men. She was not used to having sexuality become a factor in her relationships. Both George and Jane learned how to overcome these fears. George and I talked about the fact that his weight loss would not make him a small person: He was still 6-feet-2-inches tall. He was still big. Also, if he had important things to say, people would still notice him. Instead of being bearlike, he could now focus on being forceful and powerful. Force and power could come from what he was saying, instead of his size.

Jane also realized that it was perfectly reasonable to have to adjust to a new way of relating to men. Her adjustment focused on the issue of control. Jane came to realize that she could *decide* when and how to get sexually involved with the men who approached her. Just because someone looked at her or approached her differently, she did not have to act differently. Jane could respond in many ways to these approaches. She began viewing the approaches as positive signs of her improved health and self-esteem. Jane and I also discussed the possibility that she may have kept men at a greater distance when she was overweight to avoid rejection. Men could sense that and would then avoid her. Perhaps now that she felt better about herself, she was more open to a different kind of communication from men. This awareness helped Jane to stay aware of her own ability to control these more sexual approaches. This awareness helped Jane continue to concentrate on weight loss. She persisted at staying healthy. Her binge eating decreased a lot. She stopped retreating into pints of chocolate ice cream, which was her way of coping with anxiety. Jane began exercising consistently again and losing weight again.

### Lifestyle Change

**Thoughts and feelings**   This stage describes the ultimate goal for weight controllers. Individuals in this difficult-to-reach stage seem *confident, but aggressively self-protective.* They are unwilling, and adamantly so, to return to a stage in which they are "mindless" about their eating, exercise, and weight. They carefully observe their eating and exercising. They become very aware of changes in their moods, routines, relationships, work, and anything else that might trigger poor food choices or overeating. They feel confident about their knowledge of weight control; of what works and what does not. Their eating and exercising patterns seem less tied to emotions than they used to be. When eating or exercising problems emerge, they view these lapses as problems to be solved. They do not view problematic eating or exercising as weaknesses in their personalities or as reasons to give up.

**Behaviors**   Weight controllers in Lifestyle Change carefully monitor their eating and weight. They weigh themselves regularly even if they had a "bad day" or a "bad week." They handle stressful situations directly without using food as a major method of coping. They enjoy eating and find eating calming and relaxing. They even eat more then they would like to occasionally. However, they almost never overeat high-fat or very sugary foods. They also actively seek healthful eating and exercise opportunities, even when their lives are disrupted by travel, vacations, or illness.

**Example**   John nearly died one day about three years ago. He went into a diabetic coma and was revived in the emergency room at a major hospital. John was very overweight and quite unaware of the toll this weight took on his body. This dramatic moment helped John stay extremely committed to change. He had a lot to live for in his work, relationships, and all aspects of his life.

John experienced the usual Honeymoon stage, followed by some frustrations. He finally settled into Lifestyle Change after approximately two years. When he got there, he was remarkably strong and focused. His eating and exercising remained consistent and consistently effective, despite frequent traveling and other disruptions. While he occasionally ate more than he wanted to, he never came close to giving up. He would increase his monitoring and rededicate himself to exercise when he found his weight moving up the scale by even two or three pounds. John lost 72 pounds and has kept virtually all of the weight off over the past three years.

Sarah also achieved the unusual status of the Lifestyle Change stage. She did not have any dramatic health problems or other crises in her life. However, she had been battling weight problems since she was a teenager. After losing approximately 30 pounds during the first year of her effort, Sarah stayed involved in group therapy that was oriented toward weight control. She maintained this involvement for four years, during which time she lapsed occasionally. She went in and out of the Frustration and Tentative Acceptance stages. However, she eventually became a very committed exerciser (after "never sweating in my life"). She now clearly prefers lower fat and lower calorie foods. She views deviations from her usual style of eating and exercising as problems, not as horrible catastrophes or crises.

Even though John and Sarah became very successful at weight control, they did not feel in complete control of the problem. They realized that their biologies were relentless and that it takes a consistent effort to maintain substantial weight losses. Neither John nor Sarah reached the exact number on the scale that they wanted to reach when they began their weight loss efforts. However, they did get into much healthier weight ranges than they had been in. They learned to accept the limitations of their bodies. They developed a peaceful sense of resolve about persistence at weight control. The emphasis here is on peaceful, not necessarily blissful.

## Persisting Through Challenging Stages

You can see that two of the secondary stages, Shock and Ambivalence and Fear of Success, are troublesome. These stages may reduce persistence or eliminate successful persistence by some individuals. If you find yourself in such a stage, remember that you *can* work your way out of it. Some ways of doing this are discussed in Chapter 7, "Taking Control: Improving Self-Control," and Chapter 8, "Stress and Coping." For now, please understand that no one develops persistent weight control in a straight line. You may get into a Honeymoon stage that lasts several weeks, or several months, or even a year. Problems emerge along the way. If you really understand that these problems, distractions, and discouraging moments occur for everybody, perhaps you will work harder to get through them and get through them faster.

Are you currently in one of the stages of change? To help you answer this question, let's consider several additional examples. Three individuals, Michael, Susan, and Janet, are described in the following pages. Several time periods are listed on the left side of the page and descriptions of their behaviors, thoughts, and feelings are presented in the middle of the page. A space is left on the right side of the page for you to identify the stage that best fits the descriptions for each of the time periods listed. My answers are shown at the end of this exercise.

Michael, Susan, and Janet experienced weight control in different ways and at different times during their efforts. How did your choices for their stages compare to mine? Did this exercise help clarify your understanding of your own stage of change? Part of the purpose of this exercise is to illustrate that frustrations are common and also commonly overcome with continued effort. In the graph shown after the descriptions, you can see that many weight controllers experience several stages of change as they pursue persistence. The three primary stages seem to be experienced by most weight controllers during their first two years. These stages include the Honeymoon, Frustration, and Tentative Acceptance stages.

You can expect to experience these stages and perhaps some others while pursuing effective weight control. As you saw in the examples of Michael, Susan, and Janet, the Honeymoon stage includes a very positive and consistent effort at change. The Frustration stage is difficult to handle; however, it seems less devastating when compared to the Shock/Ambivalence stage (as the example of Michael illustrates). Most weight controllers spend a fair amount of time in Frustration. It is a struggle to accept the challenges, to accept the biological resistance, and to persist in the face of lapses and other distractions. If you manage to "hang in there" through your Frustration stages, you can expect to reach Tentative Acceptance. Tentative Acceptance includes a peaceful sense of resolve about the process of change. People in this stage feel that they have a clear direction about how to handle their challenging biologies. They also have refined their knowledge of nutrition and exercise and no longer struggle as much to live with the demands required for success.

The less common secondary stages include Lifestyle Change. This is the ideal or ultimate goal for weight control. Unfortunately, relatively few people actually get there. However, many weight controllers develop the aggressive self-protectiveness that characterizes this stage. They adopt this attitude even though they generally "live" somewhere in between Frustration and Tentative Acceptance.

| Time (months) | Description | Stage |
|---|---|---|
| **Michael** | | |
| 0–2 | Michael was incredibly eager to embrace all of the ideas presented in his program. He participated in a professionally conducted program designed to help people improve their abilities to focus and modify their eating and exercising habits. He was a very attentive group member, and he also completed every possible task presented to him on time and in great detail. His recording of his eating (self-monitoring) was impeccable. Michael gradually increased his daily exercising from a 5-to-10-minute walk to a 45-minute fast walk. He lost one to three pounds almost every week | _____ |
| 3 | Quite unexpectedly, MIchael began missing group sessions. His eating records became spotty and he began complaining about the demands of the program. He reported substantial binges that occurred several times per week. Michael discontinued his involvement in the program and did not answer either telephone or written correspondence from his group leader. | _____ |
| **Susan** | | |
| 0–13 | Susan also participated in a professional weight control program. She was approximately 120 pounds overweight, but was eager to change. She began exercising by walking and occasionally swimming. As she became more fit, she bought a treadmill for use at home. She eventually joined a health club and began lifting weights and stretching with the help of a professional trainer. Her exercising was very consistent and quite extensive. Susan reported great joy in both doing her exercising and the challenge of weight lifting. She followed a very low-calorie regimen (approximately 800 calories per day), relying on frozen dinner entrees for most of her lunch and dinner meals. This helped her keep the calorie levels well controlled. She avoided restaurants and parties and lost weight rapidly. She reported that it seemed "easy." | _____ |

14–20    Susan suffered a back injury during one of her    _____
workouts. This back injury was quickly
followed by a serious bout with the flu. These
experiences seemed to derail her. Her exercising was slowed down considerably due to the
injury and illness. Susan attempted to
reengage exercising as quickly as possible,
but had to yield to her physical limitations. Her
eating began to include binges on cookies and
other foods that are high in fat and sugar. Her
monitoring changed from perfectly consistent
to quite inconsistent. She reported great annoyance at the unfairness of her physical maladies.

21–24    Susan finally decided that this was one aspect    _____
of her life that she could control. She reiniti-
ated her monitoring on a consistent basis. Her
exercising did not go back to the level it had
been during her first year, but she became
more consistent, and varied her exercising to
accommodate her back injury. Susan talked
about feeling more committed and more willing
to face the problem of her binge eating "head
on."

**Janet**

0–1    Janet had difficulty monitoring. She understood    _____
the rationale for it completely, but she "didn't
want to face it." She avoided talking in her
Take Off Pounds Sensibly (TOPS) group.
Other TOPS members tried to encourage her
to discuss her feelings. Janet resisted. She
sometimes arrived at her group late and
seemed to fidget or read. She didn't seem to
want to be there.

2–9    Janet gradually began talking more in the    _____
group. Her discussions included emphasizing
why weight control was important to her. Her
monitoring improved dramatically. She began
losing weight consistently.

10–14    Janet took a vacation to Europe. Upon    _____
returning, she reported to her group that she
"lost her focus completely." She talked about
being around other people who didn't have to
worry about this problem. She had trouble
facing the nature of her biology and the
inherent unfairness of it. Her attendance was
consistent, but her efforts were not.

15–20    Janet began to complain less and monitor                    _____
more. Her monitoring improved in quality to
where it had been in the earlier part of her
first year of this effort. Her exercising became
quite consistent. She started talking about how
she enjoyed the way she felt after she
finished working out. She said it made her
feel better all day and much more relaxed.

21–22    Janet's weight loss slowed down considerably.              _____
She couldn't understand it. She had more
difficulty monitoring. She still maintained her
consistent attendance at groups, however. She
wished there was some easier way. She
began considering some radical alternatives.

23–24    After trying "Fast & Slim," Janet returned to              _____
her old methods. She found that her binges
seemed to increase as she attempted to stay
on the primarily liquid diet. She didn't like the
way it made her feel. She got back into a
more consistent exercise pattern. She talked
about refusing to give up. Janet also began
helping other group members cope with their
frustrating moments. She still had some
difficulties when she was sick or when she
went to visit her parents. Her food choices
were problematic in these circumstances.

*Answers:* Michael: Honeymoon, Shock/Ambivalence; Susan: Honeymoon,
Frustration, Tentative Acceptance; Janet: Shock/Ambivalence, Honey-
moon, Frustration, Tentative Acceptance, Shock/Ambivalence, Tentative
Acceptance.

## Chart Your Own Stages of Change

The graph at the bottom of the following page shows another
method of illustrating the stages of change. It charts the percentages of
time spent in the primary stages by a "typical" weight controller. This
person joined a formal weight control conducted by professional
therapists. Notice that the Honeymoon stage dominates the first 3 months.
Thereafter Frustration builds to a steady dosage. Tentative Acceptance
emerges during the second half of the year. The blank version of this
graph on page 49 allows you to enter your own data. Consider writing
in the percentage of time you spend in each stage during the next 12

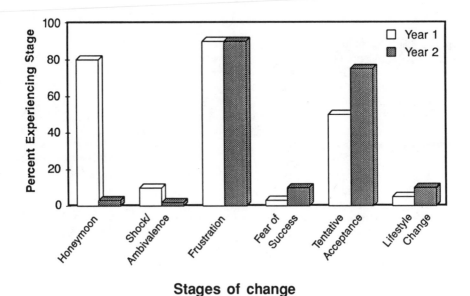

**Stages of change**

months. You will observe marked changes in your own behaviors, feelings, and thoughts as you work toward permanent change.

This model of stages of change allows you to understand what will happen to you, clarify your expectations, and improve your commitment. You now know, for example, that almost all weight controllers experience a good deal of frustration on the road to success. If you take the necessary steps to grapple with this frustration and get through it, a more peaceful,

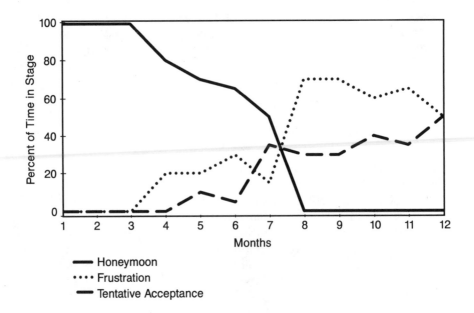

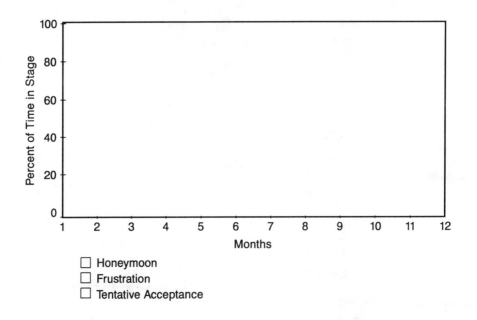

□ Honeymoon
□ Frustration
□ Tentative Acceptance

focused approach is likely to follow. You also know that most people continue to struggle, at least to some degree, with the challenges of weight control. Reaching the ultimate goal (Lifestyle Change) is not necessary for success. Persistence is necessary. As your skills in persistence improve, the struggles get easier. The rest of this book can help you improve those skills.

## Key Principles

- Expectations affect outcomes. If people expect to succeed, they often do; if they expect to fail, they rarely succeed.

- You can expect weight control to include some positive, enthusiastic times as well as some challenging, frustrating times.

- Most weight controllers experience a very positive Honeymoon stage, an annoying Frustration stage, and a more peaceful Tentative Acceptance stage.

- You can expect to spend a lot of time in both the Frustration and Tentative Acceptance stages. The clarity of focus and peaceful sense of resolve in the Tentative Acceptance stage makes it an effective place for weight controllers to be.

- Relatively few people achieve the Lifestyle Change stage. However, *aggressive self-protectiveness* that characterizes this stage is a critical goal for all persistent weight controllers. You can expect to develop that attitude if you continue to focus on your weight control efforts.

# Epilogue

## The Power of Positive Expectations

Before 1900, patients who sought medical treatment were "purged, puked, poisoned, punctured, cut, cupped, blistered, bled, leeched, heated, frozen, sweated, and shocked," according to Arthur Shapiro and Larry Morris's 1978 article in *Handbook of Psychotherapy and Behavior Change*. Irving Kirsch, in his 1990 book, noted that the "medications" prescribed by the physician in the nineteenth century and earlier included lizard's blood, crocodile dung, pig's teeth, putrid meat, fly specks, frog's sperm, powered stone, human sweat, worms, spiders, furs, and feathers. These "treatments" have been shown to have no physical properties that could lead to a cure of anything. In fact, some of them could certainly cause harm. Yet, amazingly, some people felt better after such bizarre ministrations! Our great-great grandparents must have *believed* in these treatments. Modern medicine still relies on the power of such positive expectations. The medicine of yesteryear relied exclusively on this power. Consider what you can do if you harness this force for weight control.

# 4

# Healthy Eating Ideas

"I can believe that my biology is a beast. Now, tell me how
to eat to tame it, subdue it, or better yet—kill it!"

This quote is from one of my clients, who expressed her frustration this
way a few years ago. It reflects several things that almost all weight controllers experience. First, the biology of excess weight seems beastly. The
fat cells never die; never go on vacation! Second, this client was hoping
that some style of eating could tame this beast. The search for the magical
combination of foods that can quiet or eliminate hunger has spawned
countless best sellers. Some tout healthy foods (grapefruit, popcorn,
grapes). Others promote truly ridiculous ideas—would you believe
"whipped cream" and "drinking man's" diets?—all in the guise of finding
the magical formula to tame the beast. It would be wonderful if there
were some special food or combination of foods that could make weight
control easier. Weight controllers keep searching for that formula. Books
keep making such promises, and hawkers of various potions make similar
claims: "For $19.95 get a six-month supply of AMAZING FAT-BAN
2000—plus a free necklace! Guaranteed to work!" (the necklace, that is).
   Weight controllers keep wanting someone to tell them where to find
the magic. The answer to this quest was actually discovered at the turn
of this century by L. Frank Baum in his masterpiece, *The Wizard of Oz*.
Baum's Dorothy came to a crucial realization only at the end of her long
journey to Oz. She finally realized that she already had the "magic" she
had been looking for before she took her first step on the yellow brick

road in Munchkinland. That message applies here. You probably already have the knowledge that you need for your pursuit of weight control. But, just as Dorothy used those ruby slippers, perhaps you could use some "ruby slippers" to help you clarify and refine what you already know about healthy eating. This chapter and the next one are designed to fortify you for the next, most difficult steps: using that knowledge to persist at changing.

## The Basics

### Energy Balance and Hunger

When the earliest humans first stood up two million years ago and looked around at each other, they saw no overweight people. These early hominids spent their days hunting and gathering. In fact, 99 percent of human history has been spent as hunters and gatherers. Only in the last 10,000 years did farming develop, and agricultural societies even today still suffer food shortages almost every year. Our ancestors, including our relatively recent ancestors from the past several thousand years, did not know the meaning of the concept "diet." Very, very few of them were overweight.

During the past few generations, however, in industrialized societies, things changed. Suddenly—very suddenly, from an evolutionary perspective—people were no longer hunting and gathering or working in the fields all day. They began sitting around more; they sat down when they worked in factories and offices; they began enjoying the luxury of sitting down for most of their days. Unfortunately, our hunter-gatherer biologies have not adapted to this luxury. Bodies are made to move—to move a lot—for most of the day. In societies where people still move around throughout the day (China, for example), obesity remains a very unusual problem. By contrast, the increase in sedentary lifestyles and proliferation of "modern conveniences" mean that many people today expend far less energy than they take in.

#### Hunger for Hunter-Gatherers

Losing weight requires a "negative energy balance." That is, to lose weight, you must take in less energy than your body expends. To maintain weight, intake must equal expenditure. Unfortunately, your body does not appreciate tinkering with the energy balance equation. Your body still functions like the bodies that hunted and gathered 2 million years ago; it provides strong urges to correct an imbalance in energy supply. When you eat less than you are accustomed to eating, or when you expend more energy than you are accustomed to expending, you get hungry. When you are very hungry, you get almost desperate to find more food and to expend less energy. *Homo erectus* did this 2 million years ago. You

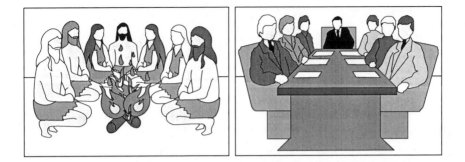

## Hunter-Gatherers

still do it today. These ancestral humans never tried to manage their hunger or to tolerate it; they just tried to satisfy it. That is the normal way to cope with hunger, the way it was meant to be. By contrast, as a weight controller, you must find ways to oppose this strong biological urge. To lose weight, you must *manage* hunger, not feed it.

### Hunger for Twentieth Century Weight Controllers

This book is devoted to helping you understand and manage feelings that people sometimes label as "hunger." Hunger can be defined in many different ways. Sometimes people define it in terms of the amount of food eaten over a given period of time. Others define it as a desire for food. The term "appetite" is also used to describe the desire for food. Here, hunger is defined as a desire for food. The following factors influence the amount or intensity of hunger:

- Biology
- Emotions
- Time of day and usual routines
- Sugar and protein consumption
- Presence of foods, particularly highly appealing and attractive foods
- Talking about food
- Thinking about food
- Eating by others
- Drinking alcohol and using other recreational drugs
- Exercise and lack of exercise

- Negative thoughts

- Variety, blandness, or strictness of diet

- Stimuli associated with eating

This list of 13 factors indicates how complicated it can be to understand your own hunger. For example, many of my clients say, "I don't eat because I'm hungry." How do they know that? When so many factors contribute to the desire for food, how can you decide when hunger motivates eating? For example, neither overweight people nor thin people can accurately determine when their bodies show certain signs of hunger, such as stomach movements. In addition, people are usually unaware of the degree to which the time of day and their usual routines affect their desire for food. If you usually snack as soon as you get in the house at the end of the work day, then coming into the house becomes a powerful trigger for eating. This is part of hunger. In addition, certain types of food (in particular sugar) can actually increase your appetite for more of the same type of food, as discussed later in this chapter. For now, you probably can identify times when eating sugary foods (like a candy bar or an ice cream cone) seem to increase your hunger rather than satisfy it.

Just talking or thinking about food can produce biological reactions in overweight people that their thinner peers never experience. One of my clients made this point beautifully. Andrea had a husband who had a "thin biology." That is, he could eat almost whatever he wanted and not gain weight. Andrea, by contrast, constantly battled her biology to maintain a reasonable weight. One day, as Andrea and her husband, Jim, were driving on the highway, Andrea noticed a truck going by that had pictures of bakery goods on the side. She pointed it out to Jim. "Hey, Jim, look at that truck over there."

Jim looked and said, "So?"

"Does that bother you or affect you in any way, seeing that truck?"

"No, of course not. Why would that bother me?"

"You see, this is exactly what I've been talking about. When I see that bakery truck with those rolls, muffins, and doughnuts, I want to eat."

"But we just had breakfast!"

"That doesn't matter!" said Andrea. "That's just the kind of biology I have. You see that truck and it's just a truck. I see that truck and I want to eat what's on it. That's the difference between us."

Hunger is also affected by exercise. Moderate amounts of exercise can decrease hunger, but remaining sedentary can increase hunger. Another factor, eating extremely bland or strict diets, can also increase binge eating and hunger. A very recent study by Christy Telch and Stewart Agras emphasized this point. These researchers found that even people who rarely binged began binge eating several times per week after completing a 12-week liquid fast.

Drinking alcohol or using other recreational drugs can change desires for food, as well. Consider the example of Carol, one of my clients. Carol kept good records of her eating and exercising usually on 5 or 6 days per week. Her records showed an excellent effort to keep her calories and the fat content of her diet very well controlled (about 1000 well-balanced, 10 percent fat calories per day). She exercised almost every day by walking several miles each morning or using a treadmill after work at a health club adjacent to her office. But mysteriously she was not losing weight despite this ostensibly flawless performance. It turned out that the day or two per week when her self-monitoring was incomplete told a lot of the story. Carol often joined her colleagues after work on Friday for an end-of-the-week celebration at a sports bar. She had a glass or two of wine (after not eating much all day) and then got into a "who cares" attitude about nibbling on bar food (peanuts, chips, barbequed chicken wings). Without the influence of alcohol, Carol knew that *she cared* about her weight control. After drinking some wine, she allowed the situation, her biological desire for food, and other factors to change her thinking and behaving.

Alcohol, marijuana, and other drugs can loosen restraints just enough to make effective weight control even more challenging than it already is. Many weight controllers do perfectly well with a glass of wine during an occasional dinner. You can observe your own patterns to determine if you have a problem like Carol's or if you can incorporate wine or other drinks into your eating/and drinking plan comfortably.

All these factors also combine in complicated ways to affect hunger. For example, traveling affects routines and emotions. Many people find traveling stressful, and it is bound to disrupt their usual routines. This may lead to eating far more calories than usual or eating more problematic foods. Part of this problematic pattern occurs due to changes in hunger. So, do you eat "when you are hungry" or not?

The point of this discussion is to emphasize the very real and powerful role of hunger in affecting your eating habits. When trying to lose weight, you place your body into a state of negative energy balance; that is, your intake can no longer meet the demands of your energy expenditures. This is the only way to lose weight. It is a type of starvation. The human body has been programmed for almost two million years to resist this state of negative energy balance. Hunger is part of that resistance. The many factors that affect hunger affect everyone who tries to lose weight.

### Charting Your Hunger

You may find it helpful to examine your own levels of hunger more systematically than you have in the past. The following pages contain forms that you can use to graph the intensity of your hunger four times per day for one week. This is a challenging task. Most people have difficulty following through with an entire week of record keeping like this. Perhaps you can use one of the day's charts to examine the intensity of your hunger during the past hours. That is, why not take a few minutes now to complete the graph for today. Can you identify clear patterns? If not, try to complete tomorrow's and the next day's hunger records. If you identify particular periods of time that you seem most hungry, that may help you cope with the hunger state more effectively. You might, for example, find that a snack in the late afternoon reduces the intensity of your hunger. You might also find that on days that you eat breakfast, you experience less hunger throughout the day than on days you skip breakfast. (This is a very common and well-established finding in scientific literature.) You will find that many of the ideas presented throughout this book can help reduce hunger. You may wish to come back to your "Weekly Hunger Record" as a means of studying the effects of some of the ideas in the book.

## Food Groups and Pyramid Power

Hunger is affected not just by how much you eat, but by what you eat as well. Most people know that eating a balanced diet provides many health benefits and avoids many health problems. The question is, "What types of food are included in this balance?" To understand the requirements for a balanced diet, it helps to understand the meaning of nutrients.

Nutrients are components of food that provide essential elements needed by your body to function effectively. You need over 45 nutrients every day. There are six classes of these nutrients that are divided into two categories: those that supply energy (calories), and those that do not supply energy. The table following the weekly records lists the six classes of nutrients needed for good health. The nutrients that supply energy, carbohydrates, proteins, and fats are most critical for weight controllers. (As discussed in the previous paragraphs, weight controllers must battle to remain in a state of negative energy balance.) However, minerals and vitamins are essential as well to sustaining life. Minerals are divided into two categories: macronutrients (those having relatively greater presence in the body) and micronutrients (those of lesser quantity, but not lesser importance, in the body). Vitamins and minerals aid in the growth of body tissue, transmit nerve impulses, regulate muscle contraction, maintain water balance, form parts of essential body compounds, maintain the acid-base balance in the cells, regulate the body's metabolism, and help transform food into energy. Fortunately, a diet that is well-balanced in

## Weekly Hunger Record

*Intensity*: Several times each day, update your graph according to the following scale:

(10) **Extremely Hungry**—I can't do anything when I'm this hungry.
(9)
(8) **Very Hungry**—My hunger makes concentration difficult, but I can perform undemanding tasks.
(7)
(6) **Hungry**—I'm hungry but I can continue what I'm doing.
(5)
(4) **Mildly Hungry**—I can ignore my hunger most of the time.
(3)
(2) **Slightly Hungry**—I notice my hunger only when I focus my attention on it.
(1)
(0) **No Hunger**

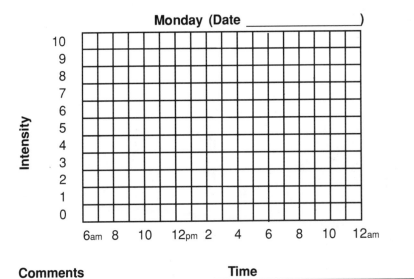

**Monday (Date _____ )**

**Comments** _____ **Time** _____

_____

_____

_____

_____

_____

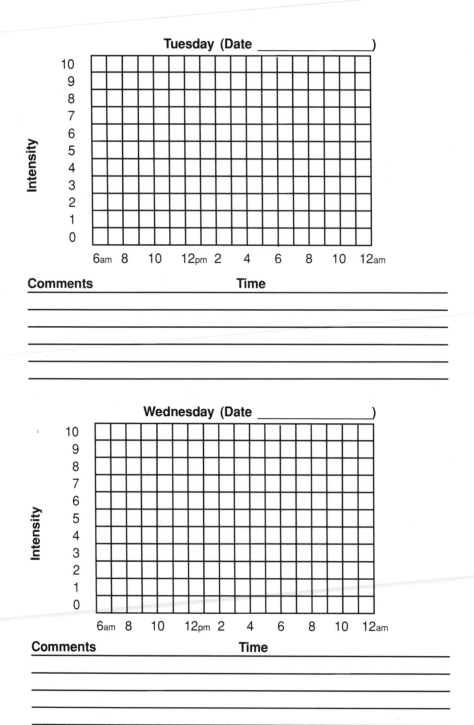

**Tuesday (Date _____)**

Intensity

10
9
8
7
6
5
4
3
2
1
0

6am   8   10   12pm   2   4   6   8   10   12am

**Comments** _____ **Time** _____

_____
_____
_____
_____

**Wednesday (Date _____)**

Intensity

10
9
8
7
6
5
4
3
2
1
0

6am   8   10   12pm   2   4   6   8   10   12am

**Comments** _____ **Time** _____

_____
_____
_____
_____

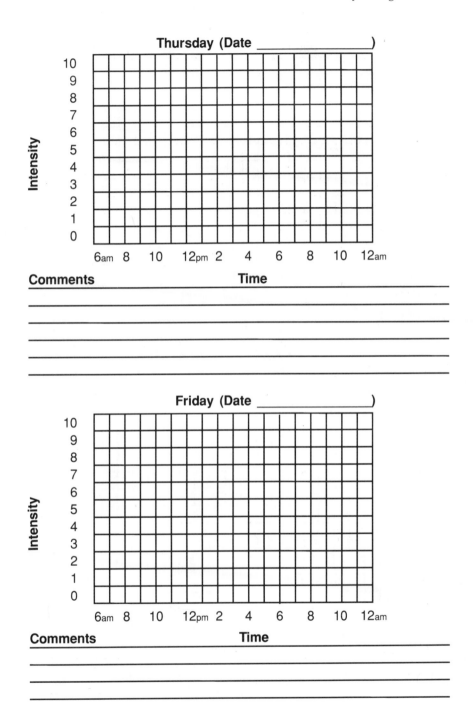

**Thursday (Date _____ )**

Intensity

10
9
8
7
6
5
4
3
2
1
0

6am   8    10   12pm  2    4    6    8    10   12am

Time

Comments _____

_____

_____

_____

_____

_____

**Friday (Date _____ )**

Intensity

10
9
8
7
6
5
4
3
2
1
0

6am   8    10   12pm  2    4    6    8    10   12am

Time

Comments _____

_____

_____

_____

_____

_____

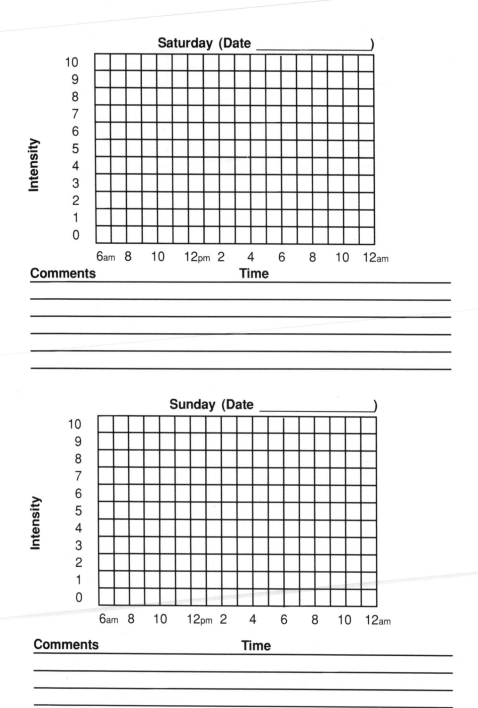

**Saturday (Date _____)**

Intensity

10
9
8
7
6
5
4
3
2
1
0

6am  8  10  12pm  2  4  6  8  10  12am

**Time**

**Comments** _____

_____

_____

_____

_____

_____


**Sunday (Date _____)**

Intensity

10
9
8
7
6
5
4
3
2
1
0

6am  8  10  12pm  2  4  6  8  10  12am

**Time**

**Comments** _____

_____

_____

_____

_____

_____

# The Six Classes of Nutrients

### Nutrients that provide energy (calories)

1. Carbohydrates: starches, sugars, and fiber
2. Proteins: includes 22 amino acids
3. Fats: saturated, monounsaturated, and polyunsaturated fatty acids

### Nutrients that do not provide energy

4. Minerals:

| *Macronutrients* | *Micronutrients* | |
| --- | --- | --- |
| calcium | arsenic | iron |
| chlorine | boron | manganese |
| magnesium | cobalt | molybdenum |
| phosphorus | copper | nickel |
| potassium | chromium | selenium |
| sodium | fluorine | silicon |
| sulfur | iodine | vanadium |
| | | zinc |

5. Vitamins:

| *Fat Soluble* | *Water Soluble* |
| --- | --- |
| A | C |
| D | $B_1$ (thiamine) |
| E | $B_2$ (riboflavin) |
| K | $B_3$ (niacin) |
| | $B_6$ (pyridoxine) |
| | $B_{12}$ (cobalamin) |
| | Folican |

6. Water

terms of various categories of food usually provides all of the essential vitamins and minerals.

To encourage Americans to eat a varied and balanced diet, and thereby consume adequate amounts of vitamins, minerals, and fiber, the U.S. Department of Agriculture officially launched the Food Guide Pyramid in 1992,which is shown below.

The pyramid graphically presents five food groups, with the grain group (bread, cereal, rice, and pasta) at the base. The pyramid structure illustrates that these complex carbohydrates are the foundation of a healthy diet. You can see that the U.S. Department of Agriculture (in co-operation with the American Dietetic Association) recommends 6 to 11 servings per day from the grain group; 2 to 4 servings per day from the fruit group; 3 to 5 servings per day from the vegetable group; 2 to 3 servings per day from the meat group; and 2 to 4 servings per day from the milk group. The tip of the pyramid is an "others" category, for foods that do not have enough nutrients to fit into any of the five major food groups. These foods include fats and oils, sweets, salty snacks, alcohol, other beverages, and condiments. The current recommendation is to use these foods sparingly.

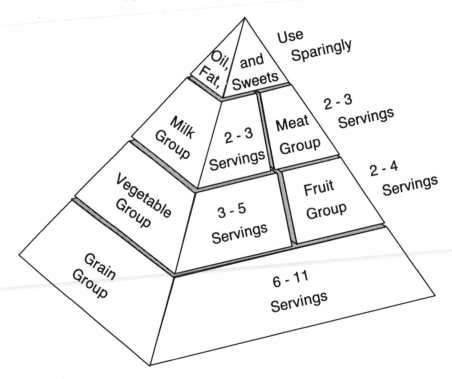

**U.S. Department of Agriculture Food Guide Pyramid**

The following sections describe the contents of a serving for each of the five food groups with some examples of recommended foods for each.

### Milk Group: 2 to 3 Servings

One serving equals 1 cup of milk or yogurt, 1 1/2 ounces of natural cheese, or 2 ounces of processed cheese. Good examples are:

- Skim and 1 percent low-fat milk
- Buttermilk made with skim or 1 percent low-fat milk
- Yogurt made with skim or 1 percent low-fat milk
- Low-fat or dry curd cottage cheese (1 to 2 percent)
- Cheeses with 2 or fewer grams of fat per ounce
- Frozen dairy desserts with 2 grams of fat or less per item or per 1/2 cup serving

### Meat Group: 2 to 3 Servings

One serving equals 2 to 3 ounces of cooked lean meat, fish, or poultry; 1 to 1 1/2 cups of cooked dried beans; 2 to 3 eggs; and 4 to 6 tablespoons of peanut butter. Good examples are:

- Beef: eye of round, top round, low-fat beef products
- Veal: all cuts except loin, rib, and ground
- Chicken or turkey without skin
- Poultry cold cuts with up to 1 gram of fat per ounce
- All fresh fish and shellfish; canned fish, water-packed, drained
- All dried beans, peas, and lentils
- Egg whites and low-fat egg substitutes

### Vegetable Group: 3 to 5 Servings

One serving equals 1 cup of raw, leafy vegetables; 1/2 cup of other vegetables (cooked or chopped raw); or 3/4 cup of vegetable juice. Good examples are:

- All fresh vegetables or frozen vegetables without sauce
- Canned vegetables
- Vegetable juices

### Fruit Group: 2 to 4 Servings

One serving equals 1 medium apple, banana, or orange; 1/2 cup of chopped, cooked, or canned fruit; 3/4 cup of fruit juice. Good examples are:

- All fresh fruit (except avocados and olives)
- Unsweetened applesauce
- Dried fruit
- Canned fruit in its own juice

### Grain Group: 6 to 11 Servings

One serving equals 1 slice of bread; 1 ounce of ready-to-eat cereal; or 1/2 cup of cooked cereal, rice, or pasta. Good examples are:

- Bread, bagels, pita, English muffins, rolls with 2 or fewer grams of fat
- Air-puffed popcorn, pretzels, rice cakes, bread sticks, corn tortillas
- Crackers with 1 gram or less of fat per 1/2 ounce: Melba toast, matzoh, flat bread, saltines
- Cold cereals with 2 or fewer grams of fat and 6 or fewer grams of sugar per serving (for example, Cheerios, Shredded Wheat, Grape Nuts)
- Hot cereals
- Rice, barley, bulgur wheat, couscous, kasha
- Pasta
- Low-fat pancakes and waffles

If your eating plan follows the guidelines provided by the pyramid, you probably will not benefit from taking vitamin or mineral supplements of any kind. You can also see by the examples provided in the previous sections that many low-fat, low-calorie foods can be used to create a balanced meal plan.

### Fiber

The pyramid guidelines also lead to a diet that is high in fiber. Fiber is defined as the part of food (plants) that cannot be broken down by enzymes in the digestive tract. Most nutritional experts endorse the National Cancer Institute's recommendations that Americans eat 20 to 35 grams of fiber per day. Most Americans currently consume less than half of that amount. The following table lists examples of various foods and their fiber contents:

| Food | Serving Size | Fiber (grams) |
|------|--------------|---------------|
| *Breads* | | |
| Rye | 1 slice | 2.0 |
| Whole wheat | 1 slice | 1.9 |
| White | 1 slice | 0.4 |
| *Cereals* | | |
| All-Bran or 100% Bran | 1 cup | 23.0 |
| Grape Nuts | 1/3 cup | 5.0 |
| Rolled oats, dry | 1/2 cup | 4.5 |
| Shredded Wheat | 2 biscuits | 6.1 |
| *Fruits* | | |
| Apple (with skin) | 1 small | 3.0 |
| Applesauce | 1/2 cup | 1.7 |
| Banana | 1 medium | 1.8 |
| Cantaloupe, cubes | 3/4 cup | 1.4 |
| Cherries, raw | 10 | 0.8 |
| Grapefruit | 1/2 | 2.6 |
| Grapes, raw | 16 | 0.4 |
| Orange | 1 small | 1.8 |
| Peach, raw | 1 medium | 1.3 |
| Plum, raw | 2 small | 1.6 |
| Strawberries | 1/2 cup | 2.6 |
| Fruit juice | 1/2 cup | 0.5 |
| *Vegetables* | | |
| Beans, green | 1/2 cup | 1.2 |
| Broccoli, cooked | 3/4 cup | 1.6 |
| Carrots, raw | 1 medium | 3.7 |
| Celery, raw | 1 stalk | 1.2 |
| Corn kernels | 2/3 cup | 4.2 |
| Cucumber | 1/2 or 7-inch | 1.5 |
| Dried peas, beans | 1/2 cup | 6.9 |
| Lettuce | 1 cup | 0.8 |
| Potatoes, cooked | 2/3 cup | 3.1 |
| Rice, white, cooked | 1 cup | 0.4 |
| *Meat, Fish, Eggs, Milk, Cheese* | | |
| All | | 0 |

Generally, diets that are high in fiber improve digestive processes and probably prevent the development of certain cancers (such as colon cancer). Fiber softens stools, reduces constipation, and speeds wastes through the intestines. This may lessen the chance that the small amounts of cancer-causing substances found in foods and produced through digestion come in contact with the surface of the colon. Eating foods that are high in fiber can also lower levels of sugar in the bloodstream, which may reduce hunger. Some fibers can also lower cholesterol levels.

Unfortunately, it is difficult to count grams of fiber in the diet. This makes it hard to determine the amount of fiber you consume. It seems wise simply to follow the general advice that encourages everyone to eat lots of fruits and vegetables every day. It also helps to choose a breakfast cereal that contains at least five grams of fiber. Eat products made from whole grains (breads, pastas) rather than refined or processed grains whenever possible, as well. Fortunately, weight controllers often find this advice relatively easy to follow as part of their efforts to lose weight.

## Water and Other Liquids

When the sweat pours off you on 90-degree summer days, you need no reminders to get something to drink. However, if you rely on thirst to tell you when to drink, you are probably drinking too little. Thirst is a signal developed through evolution to prevent severe dehydration. It only becomes active when your body is in trouble. The thirst signal also shuts off well before you have had enough to drink. Your body uses about three quarts of water a day—even if you do nothing special. The fluids within foods and liquids usually replace this loss. However, weight controllers require additional fluids due to the special demands placed on their bodies through exercise and dieting. The following are the benefits of drinking eight 8-ounce glasses of noncaffeinated fluids every day, plus an additional glass for every 25 pounds of excess weight:

- **Fluids decrease hunger naturally.** Many weight controllers drink water and other noncaffeinated beverages both before and during meals. It may also help to eat soups whenever possible. In at least one study, soups were shown to help decrease appetite.

- **High levels of fluid intake help the liver break down stored fat.** During weight reduction, the kidneys work especially hard to get rid of by-products of using the stored fat. If fluid supplies are maintained at a high level, the kidneys can function very effectively at this task. If you do not drink an adequate amount of noncaffeinated liquid, however, the liver takes over part of the kidneys' function to make sure the blood is filtered properly. If the liver has to do some of the kidneys' work, it can't operate as effectively as it normally does. Therefore, it slows down the process of releasing some of the energy from stored fat, and more fat remains stored in the body instead. This slows down weight reduction.

- **Drinking enough fluids helps reduce fluid retention.** If the body gets an inadequate amount of fluids, it operates as if its survival has been threatened. Therefore, it holds onto every drop of liquid. Water gets stored in spaces outside of the cells, and this can show up as swollen feet, legs, and hands. The single best way of ridding the body of excess fluid is to drink more liquid. If the body gets plenty of water (or other noncaffeinated liquid), it will release more water from the cells. This results in less swelling and decreased excess weight.

- **Drinking adequate amounts of fluids prevents the skin from shrinking and the muscles from becoming weak**. When you're dehydrated, you tend to feel irritable, dizzy, headachy, and drained of energy. Your muscles don't function well and your skin begins to sag. Maintaining appropriate fluid levels prevents these problems.

- **Fluids promote effective digestion.** Too little fluids often result in constipation. Adequate amounts of fluids promote normal bowel functioning. This could also decrease the risk of colon cancers.

The benefits to drinking adequate amounts of fluids are clear. This is very important for all weight controllers. It also helps to drink cold liquids that have little or no caffeine in them. You might be wondering why only noncaffeinated drinks are recommended. One cup of brewed coffee contains approximately 11 milligrams of caffeine. Tea contains approximately half that amount of caffeine, and colas contain approximately one-quarter of that amount. Caffeine leeches fluids from the cells (and therefore is a diuretic). There is so much caffeine in a cup of brewed coffee that drinking coffee adds essentially no liquids to your body. In a similar vein, drinking one cup of tea probably adds about the equivalent of one-half cup of water. Caffeinated colas add about three-quarters of a cup of fluid intake for every full cup drunk.

It is important to replace fluids lost during exercise as well. You may not be aware of the perspiration that you lose when you exercise. Remember, your body cools itself by sweating. When your muscles work hard and when you breathe rapidly, you lose fluids whether you notice it or not. For example, the little water droplets that create the "smoke" you exhale on very cold days demonstrate that you exhale water as well as carbon dioxide. For every pound that you lose when you exercise, it helps to drink one pint (16 ounces) of noncaffeinated fluid. It is particularly helpful to replenish the lost fluid within one-half hour of exercising. Drinking cold liquids soon after exercising helps your body absorb them most readily. You do not have to consider replacing the salt lost by sweating unless you have lost ten pound during an exercising session. Also, drinks that are heavily promoted as "sports drinks" contain sugar and salt, neither of which is helpful for most weight controllers.

## Problematic Foods

The following table lists six potentially harmful foods and nutrients and the problems associated with them,. The two items that produce the greatest problems for people interested in losing weight are fat and sugar.

### Potentially Harmful Foods and Nutrients

| Food or Nutrient | Potential Problems |
|---|---|
| *Cholesterol* (the "bad" kind, low-density lipoproteins): A fatty substance, part of fat contained in animal tissue; contained in all animal products, especially egg yolks and organ meats like liver | Can raise levels of cholesterol in blood, which can increase risk of heart disease and strokes; may contribute to risk of colon, breast, or prostate cancers. |
| *Fat:* Fatty meats and fish, butter, vegetable oils, eggs, cheeses, pastries | Saturated fats (mostly those that are solid at room temperature) raise levels of harmful cholesterol in blood (see effects above); high consumption of all fats increases risk of colon and probably breast and prostate cancers. |
| *Nitrite-cured or smoked foods:* Bacon, hot dogs, sausage, bologna, salami, smoked fish. | May increase risk of stomach and esophagus cancers. |
| *Salt:* Table salt, many processed foods, including soups, canned vegetables, fast foods, salt-cured foods | Can raise blood pressure to high risk levels in some individuals; thereby increasing risk of heart disease and stroke. |
| *Sugar:* Refined sugars in candies, pastries, cakes, most breakfast cereals; natural sugars in fruits, honey, milk, and sweet alcohols | Increases tooth decay, increases craving for more sugar; may contribute to irritability, excessive activity, and weight gain. |
| *Alcohol:* Liquor, wine, beer | At high intake, greatly increases risk of liver diseases, increases likelihood of car accidents even in moderate doses, and can increase blood pressure. |

## Fat Begets Fat

"Any pig farmer knows that you can't get pigs fat feeding them wheat; you need corn, which contains more oil," says Professor Elliot Danforth. Danforth and his colleague, Ethan Allen Sims, professors at the University of Vermont, studied the effects and causes of obesity. Using male prisoners as subjects, they asked the prisoners to eat large amounts of food and then observed the effects. They found that the prisoners who ate a lot of high-fat foods gained weight much more easily than those who ate foods that were lower in fat and higher in carbohydrates. More recent studies also show that high-fat foods are most easily stored as additional fat in the body. For example, to turn 100 calories of very high-fat food like butter or bacon into body fat, your body only expends about 3 calories of energy. That means that 97 calories of the 100 calories end up in your fat cells. Turning carbohydrates into fat is much more complicated. The body has to change the carbohydrate into a number of other chemical compounds in order to process it. As a result, in order to turn 100 calories of spaghetti into fat, the body has to expend about 23 calories. In other words, it costs a lot of energy to transform foods that already start out as fat into body fat. Therefore, 100 calories of spaghetti may translate into 77 calories of fat, whereas 100 calories of butter transforms into 97 calories of fat.

Overweight (and formerly overweight) people have additional reasons to avoid eating fat. People who struggle with their weight have more of the enzyme lipoprotein lipase (LPL) in their bodies than never-overweight people. When normal people eat fat (like bacon or butter), their bodies lower their LPL levels. This response helps them use the fat for energy right away, instead of storing it in the fat cells. When obese or formerly obese people eat bacon or butter their LPL levels soar to new heights! This response enables their bodies to store the fat into their fat cells very quickly. As Trudy Yost, an obesity researcher, put it recently, "These bodies are preferentially pulling fat calories out for storage." The moral is: Avoid foods that are high in fat.

### How Low Can You Go?

Is it helpful for weight controllers to eat very little fat, no fat, or somewhere in between? First, to answer this question, you need to know how to measure the amount of fat in your diet. The most effective way to calculate fat in your diet is to determine the percentage of the total calories you consume that comes from fat. The table on potentially harmful foods indicates that certain types of fat (in particular, saturated fats) create more health problems than other types of fat (for example, monounsaturated fats, such as olive oil and peanut oil). This is certainly true. However, from a weight control perspective, a fat is a fat is a fat. In other words, all fats contain approximately the same number of calories. And all fats are stored by your body as fat very readily. In this respect:

peanut oil = lard = corn oil = coconut oil

So, the question of greatest concern to those who want to lose weight is, "How much fat am I eating," not "What kind of fat am I eating."

To calculate the percentage of your calories that comes from fat, first you must know the total number of calories you consume for a particular day. Then you will want to determine the number of fat grams you consumed. You can use simple arithmetic to translate the number of fat grams eaten per day to the percentage of calories consumed that day from fat. Consider the examples presented here:

### Chicken Sandwich

| Ingredients | Calories | Fat Grams |
|---|---|---|
| Chicken (3 ounces) | 142 | 3 |
| Light wheat bread (2 slices) | 80 | 1 |
| Lettuce (1 leaf) | 3 | 0 |
| Tomato (2 slices) | 12 | 0 |
| Mustard or no-fat mayonnaise (1 teaspoon) | 8 | 0 |
| Apple (1 medium) | 80 | 1 |
| Diet coke or iced tea | 0 | 0 |
| Total calories = | 325 | |
| Total fat grams = | | 5 |

*Number of fat grams x number of calories per gram (9) = calories from fat:*
    5 x 9 = 45

*Percent calories consumed from fat = calories from fat divided by total calories:*
    45/325 = 14%

### McDonald's Big Mac Meal

| | Calories | Fat Grams |
|---|---|---|
| McDonald's Big Mac | 572 | 34 |
| McDonald's fries (small) | 222 | 12 |
| McDonald's chocolate shake | 356 | 10 |
| Total calories = | 1150 | |
| Total fat grams = | | 56 |

*Number of fat grams x number of calories per gram (9) = calories from fat:*
    56 x 9 = 504

*Percent of calories consumed from fat = calories from fat divided by total calories:*
    504/1150 = 44%

The McDonald's Big Mac meal certainly outweighs (outfats?) the chicken sandwich meal in all ways. The McDonald's meal includes approximately 4 times as many calories and 11 times as much fat as the chicken sandwich meal. These examples show more than these obvious differences between these choices for lunch. Very few weight controllers choose McDonald's Big Mac meals as the mainstay of their diets. However, this meal, as well as the chicken sandwich meal, illustrate that measuring the amount of fat in your diet requires attention to the number of fat grams consumed and the total number of calories consumed. Actually, if you keep records of your total consumption of food and total fat gram consumption for a day, then you can calculate the percentage of fat in your diet.

Some recent studies indicate that obese people tend to get higher percentages of their calories from fat than lean people do. Some obese people eat similar numbers of total calories compared to non-obese individuals, but the percentages of fat in their diets can be 25 percent higher than non-obese people. If you want to lose weight, you must consume very low percentages of fat in your meal plans. The American Heart Association suggests that if Americans adopted a diet consisting of 30 percent of calories from fat, there would be much less heart disease in this country. Right now Americans consume closer to 40 percent of their total calories from fat. Reducing to diets containing 30 percent fat would surely improve the health of many people; but this level is still too high for people who wish to lose weight. Most experts recommend that a better percentage for weight controllers is 20 or 25 percent. My recommendation is even simpler than that. I encourage you to consume as low a percentage of your total intake from fat as you can tolerate. So, the answer to the question, "How low can you go?" is, "As low as possible!" For most people, this means aiming for 10 to 20 percent of calories consumed as fat.

Living with a very low-fat eating plan presents many challenges. This is the age of motorized dessert carts and specialty cookie shops on every street corner. While people talk about exercising more than ever before, many people exercise on their way to fast food restaurants (like the President, Bill Clinton). Others enjoy wearing the clothing of exercisers; but participating is a different story. The same applies to living life without high-fat foods. For example, in an October 1992 *Consumers' Report* article entitled "Are You Eating Right?," the editors noted that Americans were "still saying 'cheese'." That is, "Americans have soured on whole milk in the past 25 years and now choose low-fat milk more often. But consumption of high-fat cheeses has more than doubled in the same period, and even cream is rising."

Despite Americans' tendency to eat high-fat foods, many people eat very few foods that are high in fat. In fact, all successful weight controllers consume much less fat in their eating plans than do average Americans. This means that successful weight controllers rarely eat red meat, hardly ever eat desserts other than fruit or low-fat/no-fat alternatives, and almost never eat any fried foods. Their salad dressings are almost always low-fat or low-calorie, and when they order salads in restaurants, salad dressings are ordered on the side. They grill and broil and bake and steam foods. They insist on being served foods prepared in those low-fat ways in restaurants. Successful weight controllers rarely eat anything with gravy or sauces (other than broths and simple tomato sauces). No-fat or low-fat cheeses, ice cream, and mayonnaise are also among their possibilities. They think of cookies, brownies, cake, and candy as foods for others, not for themselves.

Many people really *can* live this way. For example, have you made the change from whole milk to skim milk? Do you miss drinking whole milk, or does whole milk seem more like cream to you now? People find some of these changes easier to implement than you might expect. For example, consider the following quotations from some of my more successful clients:

- "It's amazing, but I don't even want candy anymore. When I see candy, or people eating candy, I don't have the slightest interest in eating it."

- "I find fried foods disgustingly greasy now. Except for french fries, fried foods don't tempt me in the least. Okay, maybe onion rings tempt me a little, too."

- "This is the best time in history for living with low-fat foods. There are so many perfectly good choices."

- "I now think of high-fat foods as 'alien foods.' I say to myself, 'that stuff is for people from other worlds'."

Some ideas about foods that have helped my clients make low-fat eating more palatable include:

- Snacks: air-popped popcorn, pretzels, fruit, rice cakes, low-calorie Jell-o, low-calorie cocoa, the usual raw vegetables (the new peeled mini-carrots are especially good).

- Mustard on everything: collect, compare, and contrast many different varieties of mustards.

- Learning to love spicy foods.

- Salsa on everything: become a salsa connoisseur and collect, compare, and contrast many different varieties.

- Pasta, pasta, pasta.

- Tomato sauces: particularly low-fat versions.

- Fish, shellfish.

- Stir-fried cooking: use broths, water, minimal oil.

- No-fat cheeses: try melting them on bagels or English muffins.

- Baked potatoes with dry, 1 percent cottage cheese or very low-fat yogurt instead of sour cream.

- Soups: experiment with vegetables, beans, bones.

- Frozen entrees that specify the amount and percent of fat (limit to 20 percent of total calories): examples with 10 percent of calories from fat or less are Healthy Choice ravioli, Healthy Choice linguini with shrimp, Tyson roasted chicken, and Ultra Slim-Fast mesquite chicken.

- Canned no-fat soups.

- When you use a little oil, choose olive oil instead of the less flavorful vegetable oils.

- Heat oil before sauteing food because cold oil is absorbed more readily than hot oil.

- Avoid adding oil to marinades. Instead, brush food lightly with oil before grilling.

- Wrap fish in lettuce before baking to retain moisture. (Remove lettuce before serving—unless, of course, you love the taste of soggy, fishy lettuce!)

- To prevent yogurt from separating when heated, add one teaspoon of cornstarch for every cup of yogurt.

- Vegetable purees can thicken sauces. Mashed or pureed potatoes make a good thickener.

- To sweeten dishes without table sugar or honey, use concentrated fruit juices such as frozen orange or apple juice.

Low-fat eating is very possible. Low-fat eating can also be very tasty. On the other hand, taste sensations are often tied directly to fat content. So, no one could convince you that low-fat eating can imitate the tastes that you can get from high-fat foods. Berries do not quite match cheesecakes or chocolate mousses. Grilled swordfish may be a real treat, but it cannot match the taste of a porterhouse steak. Unfortunately, high-fat food choices must become "alien food" to you if you expect to lose weight and keep it off forever. You *can* do it. Many, many thousands of people have made the switch to low-fat eating. It becomes part of a way of life. It can be a very satisfying way of life. In any case, it beats the alternative for those of us who have lost weight. You cannot get to a lower weight and stay there without adopting a very low-fat eating plan.

## Cholesterol: Clarifying Confusions

The previous discussion mentioned cholesterol. When cardiologists talk about fat, they are particularly concerned about the build-up of cholesterol in the bloodstream. People are often confused about cholesterol. They do not understand what it is, how it is created and stored in their bodies, or the relationship between cholesterol and fat in their diets. But most people do understand that cholesterol is something to avoid. It is worthwhile to consider a bit more about the nature of cholesterol and how it can affect your health.

This discussion focuses exclusively on the health of your heart and your circulatory system. The implications of your cholesterol level are quite different from the process of losing weight and keeping it off. The connection between the two pertains only to the fact that weight control requires a substantial reduction in the amount of fat in your diet. Reducing cholesterol levels also involves avoiding certain types of fat. A point emphasized earlier in this chapter deserves a second mention here: From the standpoint of losing weight, a fat is a fat is a fat. All fats create similar problems for people who are trying to lose weight and maintain low body weights. Certain fats, however, pose special health risks because they contribute to the build-up of harmful, fatty substances in the body known as cholesterol.

Cholesterol is a waxy, fat-like substance. It is found in all animals and, therefore, in all animal products, including meat, eggs, fish, poultry, and dairy products. No foods that are derived from plants contain any cholesterol. However, just as consumption of saturated fat from animal products can raise cholesterol levels, so can consumption of other forms of saturated fat, such as tropical oils (palm and coconut) and "trans-fat" (found in stick margarines and some vegetable shortenings). Cholesterol is in all tissues in the human body (as well as in other animals), including the bloodstream. Cholesterol is essential to life. It is used to form a wide variety of vital substances, including cell membranes. The body makes all the cholesterol it needs. Cholesterol is not an essential nutrient. This means that you do not need to consume any cholesterol to stay healthy.

Your body manufactures most of the cholesterol in your bloodstream. Your body produces about a thousand milligrams a day of cholesterol. In addition, most Americans consume between 400 to 500 milligrams of cholesterol in their food. In a way, that means there are two different varieties of cholesterol. There is one kind that is derived from food (referred to as dietary cholesterol), and there is another kind that is made by the body (manufactured cholesterol).

Both dietary cholesterol and manufactured cholesterol can build up in the bloodstream. This creates potentially serious problems. This fat-like substance can accumulate in the walls of the blood vessels and interfere with the flow of blood through those vessels. When this condition becomes a significant problem, it is known as atherosclerosis. Sometimes plaques are formed. These are hardened pieces of cholesterol that decrease the flow of blood and sometimes form blood clots. These plaques may cut off the flow of blood almost completely, or completely, by getting into the arteries that nourish the heart. This is a "heart attack." Also, the accumulating cholesterol in the arteries and veins can break off and clog vessels in the brain. This causes a "stroke." A stroke is the death of a part of the brain. This causes difficulties with speech, language, and movement. If the stroke is sever enough or if a heart attack is severe enough, too little oxygen gets into the brain and the person dies.

Problems associated with high levels of cholesterol make it important for everyone to know the meaning and the amounts of their current cholesterol levels. A simple blood test can tell you the amount of total cholesterol in your bloodstream, the amount of the "good" kind of cholesterol, or high-density lipoprotein (HDL), and the amounts of the "bad" type of cholesterol, or low-density lipoprotein (LDL). (One way to remember which type of cholesterol is which, is to think of "lousy" for LDL and "helpful" for HDL.) The LDL type of cholesterol carries cholesterol through the bloodstream, dropping it off where it is needed for building cells. Unfortunately, LDL cholesterol also leaves unused residues of cholesterol in the walls of your arteries. HDL, in contrast, picks up the cholesterol from the bloodstream and the arterial walls and brings it to the liver for reprocessing or excretion. In other words, LDL brings cholesterol into the system, whereas HDL clears cholesterol out of the system.

The latest recommendations for safe levels of cholesterol have been published by the National Institutes of Health, including the National Cholesterol Education Program. The following chart shows desirable, borderline, and problematic levels of the different types of cholesterol:

| Level | Total Cholesterol (mg/dl) | LDL (mg/dl) | HDL (mg/dl) |
|---|---|---|---|
| Desirable | Less than 200 | Less than 130 | 70+ |
| Borderline | 200–239 | 130–159 | 36–69 |
| Problematic | 240+ | 160+ | Less than 35 |

Approximately 25 percent of all Americans have high cholesterol, and another 25 percent have cholesterol readings in the borderline range. If you have borderline or high total cholesterols, please consider taking steps to lower your cholesterol levels. This would be especially advisable if you have had any coronary artery disease. Also, men would be especially wise to decrease problematic cholesterol levels. Heart disease rates are three to four times higher in men than in women in middle age, and about twice as high among the elderly. In addition, if your family history includes people with heart disease, if you are a cigarette smoker, if you have high blood pressure, if you are obese, or if you have diabetes, it is especially important to take steps to improve your cholesterol levels.

The following methods can improve your cholesterol profile:

- Lose weight.

- Cut down on dietary cholesterol and saturated fats (meats, whole milk, whole milk cheeses, coconut, palm, and palm kernel oils).

- Avoid "trans-fat": vegetable shortening (partially hydrogenated oils), margarine that comes in sticks (tub margarine and diet or light margarine are much better).

- Use olive, peanut, canola, and corn oil.

- Quit smoking.

- Avoid anabolic steroids.

- Consume more soluble fiber (oats, beans, fruits, vegetables).

- Consume more fish (for their omega-3 fatty acids).

In addition, your internist could prescribe a cholesterol-lowering drug if these other methods do not produce satisfactory results. Taking these steps can substantially reduce your risk for heart disease and related circulatory problems.

## Sugar

Happiness is the reward of an active life lined with "sweet reason," according to Aristotle. Here is another quote, from "Food for Thought," by Susan Cohler:

> In the harsh light of the suburban ice cream parlor, a
> gangly adolescent creates a masterpiece. Three scoops of
> sweet delight nestled side by side, enfolded in the arms of
> a ripe banana. Steaming fudge drapes the ice cream slopes
> and snakes its way to the depths of the dish. A cloud of
> whipped cream, bejeweled with nuts and one cherry crowns
> the top. This ice cream treat is a work of edible art, but
> what it does to [you] ... may be worth thinking about.

Sugar clearly permeates our lives. Not only can sugar serve as the foundation for "edible art," it plays a major part in almost all holiday celebrations, including Valentine's Day, Easter, and Christmas. Think about the well-known phrases, "Home sweet home" and "How sweet it is!" Think of many of the most common terms of endearment: sugar, sweetheart, sweetie, cookie, honeybunch, sugar plum, and sweet pea. I have

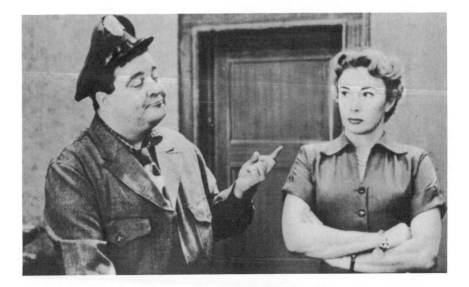

**The Honeymooners**

personally used many of these terms to refer to my two young sons. It makes me smile just to think of them with these phrases in mind, even as I write this sentence. Not only do relationships involve sugar metaphors, but so do sports performances. Have you seen a sports telecast that did *not* include such phrases as "sweet shot?" Sugar is idealized in these phrases. The best thing you could say about a person is that they are sweet.

In the 1950s' TV classic, "The Honeymooners," Jackie Gleason starred as the hapless, but lovable, bus driver, Ralph Kramden, who was always looking for an angle to get rich quick. One day, Ralph decided to take an inventory of his own "good points" and "bad points." This, he figured, would help him find a way to "make it." He could try to accentuate his strengths and minimize his weaknesses. Success would then greet him with open arms, or so he thought, anyway. His best friend and upstairs neighbor was a very goofy plumber named Ed Norton, played brilliantly by Art Carney. As Ralph began composing his inventory, Ed came in for a visit. Ralph was struggling with the list. He couldn't think of any "bad points." So he asked Ed to compose the list. Ed was glad to help, as usual. After an elaborate prewriting ritual of arm swinging, throat clearing, pencil sharpening, and knuckle cracking, Ed started to write down Ralph's "bad points." He wrote decisively, quickly, and started filling up the paper easily. Ralph became annoyed, "Come on already, Norton! I can't have that many 'bad points.' What about my 'good points'?"

Ed said, "Okay! Okay! I'm getting to that. Here we go." He wrote out "Good Points," underlined it, and read it aloud. He then wrote for two seconds, put his pencil down with a flourish, and asserted in a thick Brooklyn accent "Dere!" (translation: "There!")

"What!!" Ralph exclaimed, smacking Norton in the shoulder histrionically. "You spend an hour writing out 'bad points' and one second on 'good points'! What kind of friend are you, Norton?"

"Wait a second, Ralph, just wait a second!" demanded Norton. "Just read it." Ralph grumpily grabbed the page and read aloud:

"Good Points:

Sweetest guy in the world."

He was touched. He "sweetly" thanked his friend and proceeded to spend the next days trying to build on this strength to achieve his elusive dream. It didn't work. Nothing ever "worked" for Ralph. (But it was a wonderful, and obviously very memorable, show. It is perhaps the best example of how calling someone "sweet" can be the highest form of praise.)

What causes this infatuation with sugar? It seems that this special role for sugar in so many parts of life must come from somewhere. In fact, some biological roots may help explain this. When you are hungry, sugar provides the quickest antidote. In other words, the sugar you eat is very similar chemically to the primary source of energy in your body— glucose. Sugar is white, refined sucrose that is derived from sugarcane and beets. It is actually composed of glucose, in addition to fructose. These components are readily split apart in the small intestine by the enzyme sucrase. All other forms of sugars are also quickly digested by the body:

Lactose = milk sugar

Maltose = malt sugar

Glucose = blood sugar = dextrose

Fruit sugar = levulose; glactose

Several other factors reveal that sugar's appeal has biological roots. First, sweet foods are safe foods. This harkens back to the earlier discussion of hunter-gatherers. Can you think of any examples of wild fruits or berries or vegetables that are sweet and also dangerous to eat? Probably not. If you find something hanging from a tree and it tastes sweet, it is almost certainly safe to eat. On the other hand, sour or bitter fruits or vegetables are much more likely to be poisonous than sweet ones.

Second, when humans or other animals starve, they consistently show heightened preferences for very sweet foods. This, again, shows the body's orientation to satisfying extreme hunger and food deprivation quickly and effectively.

### Sugar Begets More Sugar

A third factor that reveals the biological roots of sugar's appeal is the body's way of increasing the craving for sugar. The graph shown below illustrates one way it does this. The graph shows that when you eat carbohydrates, especially sugar, production of insulin increases. Insulin directs glucose supplies into muscles and other organs. When you eat a sugary snack, a candy bar for example, the body reacts to it by producing an excessive amount of insulin. This probably occurs because the body is programmed to eat large amounts of sugar or sweet foods whenever they are available. This would make a lot of sense for hunter-gatherers. If they found something that tasted sweet, their bodies wanted to encourage them to eat large quantities of it. So, when you eat that candy bar, your body is over-prepared to digest it. This over-preparedness includes and excess amount of insulin that essentially clears the blood of most of its energy supply (glucose). This results in a very low level of glucose in the blood. The brain then detects this low level of glucose and causes a substantial increase in hunger. In other words, when you eat sugary foods, it creates a biochemical chain reaction leading to increased hunger. The research that supports these assertions includes studies in which rabbits were fed glucose directly into their stomachs. These rabbits then ate more, after receiving a high dose of sugar, than they did under normal conditions, and quite a bit more than rabbits who received only salt water into their stomachs. A previous section discussed how "fat begets fat." In this section, the emphasis is, "sugar begets more sugar."

Mark, a very dedicated weight controller, tried to eat all of the right things. Early on in his participation in my treatment program, I noticed that he ate muesli regularly for breakfast. Muesli, granola, and similar foods have a reputation of being health foods. After all, they are made

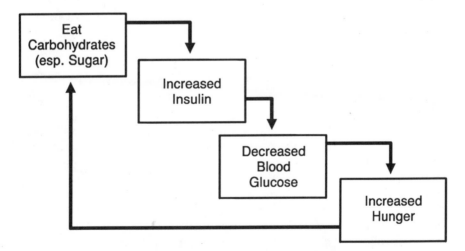

**Sugar Cycle and Weight Gain**

from whole grains, contain lots of fiber, and are sold in health food stores. Unfortunately, these breakfast cereals, as well as granola and other "breakfast" bars, contain lots of sugar. Sometimes the sugar is in the form of honey. But your body can't tell the difference between honey and sugar. Honey does contain small amounts of such minerals as potassium and calcium. But you would have to eat 200 tablespoons of honey to meet the body's daily requirement for calcium!

Mark was persuaded that his muesli wasn't great for him. So he substituted shredded wheat for muesli. he was amazed that this simple substitution resulted in much less hunger throughout the day and dramatically decreased cravings for sweets.

Recently, a new member joined the group in which Mark still participates. Linda was eating low-fat granola for breakfast regularly. She also was snacking on candy bars later in the morning and sometimes in the afternoon as well. This pattern had contributed to significant weight gain over the past couple of years. Mark and I persuaded Linda to substitute a low-sugar food for her granola. She agreed that "it's worth a shot." She began eating a bagel and low-fat cream cheese as an alternative to her usual breakfast of granola. She came back from this experiment saying, "the 'Museli Syndrome' lives! I can't believe what a difference this made. I'm also amazed that it worked immediately. As soon as I started eating bagels instead of Granola, I didn't have that gnawing feeling in my stomach anymore at ten o'clock. Wow!"

Eating sugary foods clearly increases the desire for more sugar. The obvious problems associated with managing the difficult physiology of excess weight are compounded when people eat foods that contain a lot of sugar. In addition, high-sugar diets can affect mood. These effects are not as dramatic or clear as many people believe, however. Many people think that sugar produces hyperactivity in children and "sugar blues" when sugar intake is decreased. The scientific evidence does not support these simple and exaggerated assertions. On the other hand, sugar certainly can affect moods under some conditions.

### Energy Boost: Candy Versus Ten-Minute Walks

Robert Thayer, a California State University psychologist, conducted an important study demonstrating that sugar can affect mood. Thayer compared the effects of eating a 1/2-ounce candy bar (of any type) with taking a rapid 10-minute walk. When subjects took a 10-minute walk, their tension level ratings decreased very quickly and stayed much lower than they were before taking the walk for 2 hours. In contrast, after eating the candy bar, tension levels increased over a 60-minute period and stayed high for the subsequent hour as well.

The following graphs show similar effects for ratings of "energy" levels. Subjects indicated feeling more energized for 30 minutes after eating the 1/2-ounce candy bar. However, their energy levels fell to much lower levels 1 to 2 hours after eating the candy. In contrast, when subjects took walks, their energy levels increased dramatically during the first 30 minutes. Their energy levels stayed well above their pre-walk states for 2 hours after taking the 10-minute walk. Eating candy can cause a logy or tired feeling because it stimulates the release of a natural tranquilizer in our brain called serotonin.

These findings are very important. They suggest a good alternative to eating sugary snacks in order to feel "energized." A ten-minute brisk walk can provide a much better "boost" than a candy bar. You won't find commercials encouraging people to take ten-minute walks for that "quick energy boost." You will find commercials hawking candy bars for that purpose. Now you know the truth about which works better.

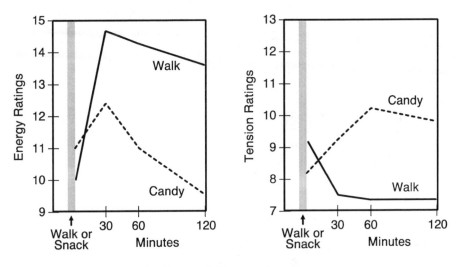

**Ratings of Energy Levels**

Sometimes even weight controllers are taken in by the advertisements and the generally positive views most people have of candy. In Margo Feiden's encyclopedic *The Calorie Factor*—675 very big pages of food listings and commentaries—she introduces candy sarcastically as "sweet little nothings." She notes: "Well, they're sweet. For the most part they're little. And as to their being 'nothings' ... " Most of my clients have found her listing of the nutritional components of candy remarkably sobering. The table below shows some of the facts behind the come-hither wrappers and ads for several of the most munched upon candies. Let the muncher beware!

Sugar can also reduce pain. Studies from researchers around the world have documented that when animals eat sugary foods they feel less pain. Eating sugary foods may release "endogenous opiates," which means that sugar can cause your body to produce its own narcotics. This probably occurs due to some biochemical reactions in the brain, but this is only speculation at this point. Elliot Blass, a psychologist from John Hopkins University, wrote an important chapter summarizing this research, "Opioids, Sweets, and a Mechanism for Positive Affect: Broad Motivational Implications." This chapter appeared in a book with an appealing title, *Sweetness*, edited by John Dobbing.

The moral of this story is: Avoid sugary foods. It is most helpful to avoid eating any snacks that contain lots of sugar, such as candy bars, ice cream cones, granola bars, caramel corn, and cookies. It is also very wise to avoid sugary breakfast cereals and all desserts other than fruit. This approach keeps the blood glucose levels relatively stable. This helps

### Candy: Gross Anatomy

| Candy Bar | Size (oz) | Cals. | Fat grams | % of Cals. from Fat |
|---|---|---|---|---|
| **Milky Way** | 3.63 | 470 | 17 | 32.6 |
| Milk chocolate, corn syrup, sugar, partially hydrogenated soybean oil, milk, cocoa powder, malt extract, whey, lactose, salt, egg whites, soy protein, artificial flavor | | | | |
| **Hershey's Kisses** | 0.16 | 24.4 | 1.11 | 41 |
| Sugar, milk, cocoa butter, chocolate, soya, lecithin, vanillin | | | | |
| **Hershey's Almond Bar (king size)** | 2.6 | 420 | 26 | 55.7 |
| Milk chocolate (sugar, milk, cocoa butter, chocolate, soya, lecithin, vanillin), almonds, tocopherols, and citric acid | | | | |
| **Snickers (king size)** | 3.7 | 510 | 24 | 42.4 |
| Milk chocolate, peanuts, corn syrup, sugar, milk, butter, lactose, salt, egg whites, soy protein, artificial flavor | | | | |

avoid some of the other chemical reactions that produce strong cravings for some very high-calorie (and high-fat) foods.

## Case History: Gail's Christmas Cookie Tradition

Gail began working with me on a major effort to lose weight six years ago. She continues attending weekly group meetings as of this writing. Gail is a 42-year-old high school teacher and a dedicated mother of two children. She had gained 50 pounds gradually over 12 years and two pregnancies during a hectic (but sedentary) life.

Gail became intensively energized during a classic Honeymoon stage six years ago. (The Honeymoon stage is one of the six stages of weight control discussed in Chapter 3.) She monitored her eating and exercising meticulously. She focused beautifully. She varied her exercising, starting with slow but consistent walking—experimenting with racquetball and swimming. She modified her eating to include primarily foods that were low in fat and sugar. Gail lapsed occasionally by eating cookies and other sweets. She took these lapses in stride and kept moving forward, persistently.

Then, six months into her honeymoon, came Christmas. "I've got to make my cookies!" she reported.

"What do you mean 'got to?'" And how many cookies are you talking about, anyway?" I asked.

"I mean I've *got to* make these cookies. It's a wonderful tradition in my family. It's one of the few traditions that my mother established when I was growing up. We all looked forward to it. It's a neat project for families. The kids design their own styles of decorating. It's creative and important. We make many batches; dozens and dozens of cookies. Then we mail them out, and give them out, as presents."

Gail certainly was committed to those cookies—to lots and lots of those cookies! Unfortunately, cookies are committed to fat cells and increasing hunger (for more cookies, especially if 200 or so are sitting around "smiling" enticingly).

Gail, her group, and I talked about this dilemma. It had no simple solution. I emphasized the biology of weight control. The group talked about using alternative artsy projects for kids. They encouraged Gail to start a new, lower calorie, tradition; they talked about spreading "the word to friends and relatives about sugar. How can words encourage people to reduce consumption of sugar (and fat), when deeds (giving the cookies) say the opposite?

Gail reacted emotionally to the idea of giving up her cookie tradition. She "couldn't" get herself to do it, she claimed. However, she did decrease the amount of cookies she and her children baked and gave away. She wound up munching on "too many cookies."

The next year Gail vacillated between the Frustration and Tentative Acceptance stages. She baked very few cookies during her third year in the program (but still munched on too many). Finally, the cookie tradition was replaced with the "artistic greeting card tradition."

Gail has lost most of the 50 pounds that she had gained over the years. She still vacillates between Frustration and Tentative Acceptance, but she spends far more time in Tentative Acceptance these days. She still munches on "too many cookies" sometimes. Her weight fluctuates more than she would like. She still persists.

## Challenging Situations

### Traveling

"When I go on my business trips to the East, I know exactly which places I like for meals and snacks. Unfortunately, most of the stuff is junk food. I know where the Pizza Huts are. I know where the Haagen-Dazs shops are. I even know where to get seemingly healthy, but high-fat, trail mixes. I seem drawn to these places when I travel. Somehow I convince myself that 'I need a break today. It's been a long, frustrating day. It's okay to eat X,Y, Z.'"

Does this sound familiar? Traveling produces many frustrations and little control. You don't know which plane is going to be late, where your luggage will wind up, and what food will be available at what times of the day. In addition, your usual patterns of eating are thrown to the wind by dehydration, jet lag, and changes in time zones. Many people also sleep less soundly when they travel. This produces yet another type of altered state. These strange internal states become juxtaposed with readily available high-fat, high-sugar foods—quite a combination!

Some of the problems when traveling and flying begin in the airplane itself. First, airplanes are kept extremely dry, as dry as the Sahara Desert! It is critical to drink at least one glass of noncaffeinated fluid for every hour you spend in flight. Consider bringing a bottle of water with you on the plane. This can improve your sense of control as it prevents dehydration. If you rely on flight attendants to get the fluid that you need, you may become both dehydrated and frustrated if they are slow or unavailable.

Another major problem that occurs when flying concerns the food. The omnipresent peanuts get 69 to 93 percent of their calories from fat. They also contain 166 calories in a 1-ounce packet. That's a lot of fat and a lot of calories in a couple of desperate gobbles. Alcoholic drinks also cause the body to lose water, exacerbating the already difficult fluid problem. They also reduce restraint or control. This can pave the way for high-calorie eating and snacking.

The in-flight meals are perhaps the most notorious problem about flying. Many of those small and sometimes very unappealing in-flight meals seem like snacks. However, they often contain 600 or more calories, many of which come from fat. The boredom of flying makes these little unappealing "snacks" seem much more appealing. Many people also think of these meals as snacks and proceed to have a full meal soon after arriving at their destinations.

Special meals provide much healthier and tastier alternatives to standard in-flight meals. These special meals are just a phone call away. Most airlines require at least 24 hours' notice, but you can't beat the price. There is no extra charge for any of the special meals. Many more people are ordering special meals now than just a few years ago. However, less than 5 percent of travelers take advantage of this important opportunity. Special meals generally have about 33 percent fewer calories and much lower percentages of fat than the standard meals. For example, United Airlines serves about 6,000 special meals per day. Their average special meal has less than 300 calories. These special meals include those that meet religious specifications (Kosher, Hindu, Moslem), diabetic, low-calorie, low-cholesterol, low-sodium, seafood plate, fruit plate, and vegetarian. That's quite a selection! I have found the seafood platters consistently good, often including crabmeat and other tasty and healthy food choices. Vegetarian meals also work well for some of my clients. One way to increase the chances of your ordering these meals on time is to ask your travel agent to include a standing order for one of the special meals. This way when you book your flights, you book your meals at the same time. Here are a few other travel tips for frequent flyers:

- If you did not order a special meal, try to minimize the fat in the standard meal. For example, as the flight attendant brings you the meal, hand him or her the margarine, salad dressing, and dessert. Simply give it to the attendant and make as minimal a comment as you would like. You are not required to justify making healthy food choices if you do not wish to.

- Remove the skin from chicken and scrape away any gravies or sauces.

- Skip the eggs, omelettes, sausages, and red meat options. Instead, select cold cereal with fruit and skim milk for breakfast and eat chicken or pasta alternatives for other meals.

- Bring low-fat snack foods with you. Raisins, crackers, cereal, and pretzels may provide good alternatives to some of the snacks available. (The tricky part is to wait until you are in the air before munching.)

- Try to plan your meals carefully on the days that you travel. For example, if you schedule a lunch or a dinner meeting when you arrive, consider turning down the in-flight meal or snack. This would be a good time to use your own low-calorie snack or request a special meal as an alternative.

Traveling by air presents many challenges, but so does traveling by car, bus, or train. All modes of travel create irregularities in schedules and moods. Many of my clients and I have found it particularly helpful to exercise in the morning before traveling. This provides some stress relief and makes it more tolerable to sit for hours on end. Another key remedy for the travails of travel is planning. That is, by carefully (even obsessively) planning your traveling, you can avoid some of the common pitfalls. Weight controllers who plan their meals carefully and ensure that low-fat, low-calorie snacks are available, for example, tend to be more successful when they travel. Weight controllers who have reached the Lifestyle Change stage often lose weight while traveling. They use traveling as an opportunity to seek out activity and to avoid the temptations of readily accessible refrigerators.

Yet another challenge imposed by traveling concerns people. Consider the following story told by Al in one of my groups:

> I am Jewish and I was born and raised in the city with big shoulders, Chicago. The city that works. Emphasis on B-I-G. My wife grew up in Memphis, Tennessee, and she's Christian. Her parents, grandparents, and all of her relatives are from the South. That's really far south—emphasis on *south*. You could say we are from different worlds—because we are.
>
> I've made huge changes in the way I eat and in the way I exercise. I've really been working at this for 3 1/2 years now and I've lost 50 pounds. I still want to lose another 50, and I'm getting there. It's a struggle every day, but I'm getting there. My wife weighs 80 pounds less than I do and eats more food and calories every day than me. Most people find that hard to believe, but it's true. She eats desserts several times per week. I almost never do. She eats fried foods occasionally, I almost never do. I exercise all the time, she almost never does. It's just the biological breaks, I guess.
>
> Well, this plays out in a pretty funny way when we go to visit her relatives in Tennessee. I don't think many of the people who live in the southern part of the United States have quite gotten into the low-fat eating business. At least my wife's relatives sure haven't. They eat ham practically for every meal! Butter, biscuits, gravy, country ham, regular ham, mayonnaise, cakes, fried everything.

I've known these fine people for more than ten years now. I've just really perplexed them in the last three. They don't know how to feed me anymore, and it presents certain challenges for all of us. For example, after we get to my wife's aunt's house, which is where we sometimes stay for weekends when we visit with her family, I immediately go to the grocery store. I stock up on skim milk, fresh vegetables, no-salt pretzels, and a few other mainstays. They've learned that I just won't eat certain things. They've made a real effort to have raw vegetables available for me and cook some foods that for them are unusual (like chicken instead of ham). They even go so far as to occasionally buy apples or some other snack food that I can eat. Unfortunately, the apples they buy don't quite meet my Chicago standards most of the time. They're usually rather anemic and bumpy. But it's a nice thought! They even avoid buttering and putting bacon fat on vegetables; quite a change for these people.

I make sure I exercise every day when I visit there. Sometimes this means getting up before my small children wake up, even if it's before the sun peeks out over the hills. This usually makes me tired, but it allows me to stay with the program in a difficult situation. Certainly these relatives try to get me to eat and they sometimes make fun of me for my "strange ways." I try not to make a big deal out of it. We seem to have adjusted to each other reasonably well.

Al effectively asserted himself with his relatives. Family members can be food-pushers. Food is a complex commodity. People use it to express themselves. Food can also be used to control situations and other people. Getting people to overeat helps some people feel less guilty about their own problematic habits. Assertiveness in food situations is discussed in greater detail in later chapters. For now, it is helpful to realize that traveling involves negotiating and asserting yourself with other people. The central question for you when you travel is: Do you have the right to eat in a healthy, effective way wherever you are? (Hint: The answer is *Yes*.)

## Holidays

Thanksgiving is a classic holiday that Americans think of as an eating orgy. Actually, in the following Thanksgiving dinner menu, you can see that many of the elements of the classic Thanksgiving meal are healthy, low-fat foods.

| Foods/Serving Size | Calories |
|---|---|
| Turkey (no skin, one-half white, one-half dark meat) - 3 oz. | 148 |
| Mashed potatoes - 1 cup | 222 |
| Gravy - 1/2 cup | 61 |
| Stuffing - 1/2 cup | 250 |
| Candied sweet potato - 1 | 144 |
| Cranberry sauce - 2 Tbsp. | 52 |
| Fresh fruit salad - 1/2 cup | 62 |
| Celery - 1 stalk | 5 |
| Carrots - 1/2 | 15 |
| Bread - 1 roll | 71 |
| Butter - 1 pat | 35 |
| White wine - 1/2 cup | 80 |
| Pumpkin pie - 1 slice | 300 |
| Whipped cream - 1/4 cup | 200 |
| Coffee | 0 |
| **Total** | **1645** |

The white meat turkey without the skin, potatoes, fresh fruit salad, celery and carrots, and even white wine pose no major problems. It's the stuffing, gravy, butter, pumpkin pie, and whipped cream that pile on the calories and the excess fat. The meal listed above derives 21 percent of its calories from fat. By selecting the low-fat components of the classic Thanksgiving dinner, you could have a perfectly satisfactory meal. My colleagues and I have found that weight controllers who are focused and plan their Thanksgiving holiday usually do quite well. Think about some of the factors here. For example, the food is predictable. The company or social aspects of the situation are predictable and possibly controllable. If you are serving the feast, you can invite people with whom you want to talk. If you are going somewhere, you can spend your time with the people whom you find interesting and enjoyable. Thanksgiving is also finite. It has a clear beginning and end. It doesn't go on and on and on for days and days with parties and parties and parties, like Christmas.

The Christmas season poses the greatest risk for weight controllers. Unlike Thanksgiving, Christmas lasts well beyond one particular day. There are the pre-Christmas parties and mini-celebrations. There are the sugary "treats" at the office. There are baking Christmas cookies and other rituals associated with high-fat, high-sugar foods. And, of course, there is an endless stream of parties that can last for several weeks, including New Year's Eve. Alcohol also flows freely during this time of the year. Many restraints are lost and replaced instead by the "holiday spirit." All of this goes on during a time of the year when the coldness of the climate in many parts of the United States makes exercising especially challenging.

Easter and other holidays pose somewhat similar problems. These holidays also involve sugary and high-fat foods, they last quite a while, and many restraints give way to the holiday spirit.

Some research indicates that many people gain several pounds during the holiday season (from Thanksgiving through New Year's). Weight controllers often gain even more weight than the average person because of their biological predispositions toward weight gain. Weight controllers can also lose the positive momentum that they may have developed prior to these holiday seasons. It is a major psychological challenge to get back into low-fat, low-sugar eating and intensive frequent exercising once you take a vacation from it. I've seen many people become derailed during the holiday season and take many months, sometimes years, to get back on track.

Several tricks of the trade have been developed by weight controllers and those who study the process. Consider the following suggestions for your holidays:

**Plan ahead.** When you plan ahead, you can predict and control your world. For example, think about your next party. Who's going to be there and what kind of food will be served? You can call your host and see what is on the menu. You can make a tentative list of what you will eat, with whom you will talk, and how you will stay focused. It is particularly important to attempt to monitor your consumption of food and calories during the holiday season.

**Avoid starvation before a celebration.** Starving before a big holiday meal often produces binge eating. Starving produces deprivation and a very strong biological response to the sight of food. This biological response includes the secretion of insulin and salvation. In other words, if you eat nothing or very little before a big holiday meal or party, you will get incredibly hungry. This reaction is more likely to lead to problematic eating than controlled eating. An alternative approach would include selecting low-fat, low-sugar foods for breakfast and lunch. Also having a small snack just before leaving for the party may help as well.

**Scope out the food scene.** After arriving, it helps to quickly survey the available options. Perhaps you will notice that there are fresh vegetables and other munchies that will work for you. You also can discern to what degree the main courses will keep you on a low-fat, low-sugar plan. This scoping may prevent you from eating high-fat snacks such as chips, dips, nuts, and party mixes.

**Use a food plan.** Once you are aware of the potential foods, it helps to develop a specific plan for what you will eat and a way of focusing on that plan. You can use a glass of diet soft drink or water to keep your attention on the conversation. You can also use this cue or some other cue (perhaps munching a raw vegetable) to remind yourself of your immediate goals and your long-range goals.

**Refocus your holiday season.** This suggestion goes well beyond an individual event or party. Holidays are traditionally focused on food and celebrations. You can break that tradition. You can focus on other people, on special projects, and on finding new creative ways to relax. Some people develop their skills in winter sports; others focus on crackling fireplaces and reading some good books.

## Restaurants

Americans ate 25 percent of their meals outside of their homes in 1975. By 1995, it is estimated that Americans will eat 50 percent of their meals outside of their homes. Restaurant meals account for almost 50 percent of every dollar Americans spend on food. Americans eat 25 percent of their restaurant meals at fast-food eateries such as McDonald's, Burger King, Wendy's, and Pizza Hut.

You probably noticed that you, too, eat more often now then ever before in your life. Restaurants offer the advantages of keeping you away from preparing food and the urge to nibble as you cook. On the other hand, restaurants often cook in mysterious ways, using more fat and more sugar than you would to prepare many meals. Some eareries can also lull you into making problematic food choices because of their style or atmosphere. In the story below, Mark Bloom describes the nostalgic allure of a famous high-fat eatery in New York, Nathan's Famous. Even though he grew up and now lives 46 miles from Nathan's, Mark Bloom finds the appeal of Nathan's very much tied in to cherished childhood memories.

I know what's good for me: fish and fowl, fresh vegetables, a decent breakfast, an apple a day—just like Mom always said. But in my dreams I still see a Nathan's Famous hot dog. I will eagerly make a 100-mile round trip to my Brooklyn chiropractor just as an excuse to stop at Nathan's Famous in Coney Island. I've been craving Nathan's hot dogs for as long as I can remember. In fact, as a child I achieved a certain status in my family for being what my parents called "a good eater." My record for a single visit to Nathan's was seven hot dogs—not counting the french fries. I was so proud.

That was in the 1950s "when eating out was so simple." [On a more recent trip to Nathan's] the seductive aroma of secret Polish spices filled the air. I leaned up against Nathan's Famous counter and ordered a hot dog—then another. Then I heard the solemn voice of the American Heart Association. "Bad for your arteries," it said.

Sure, I know that. So I promised right there to eat low on the fat scale for the rest of the week. And I did.

Many of the nation's 700,000 restaurants do not have the allure of a Nathan's Famous, but most restaurants do have food choices as high in fat as Nathan's hot dog—and plenty of them. The sauces, butter, and oil in the salad dressing, the cream and cheese in the pasta sauces, and shortening in the pie crusts make for very high-fat eating. Many restaurant foods also contain more than ample supplies of sugar. Burgers, french fries, and milkshakes have become standard lunches for many Americans. This kind of high-fat, high-sugar eating seems normal to most people. Successful weight controllers cannot and do not live that way.

Eating in restaurants can work very well for weight controllers. It requires clarity of thinking and assertiveness. Do you believe you have the right to get what you pay for? If the answer is yes, and I certainly hope it is, then it is your *right* to request that the food you order at a restaurant is prepared in accord with your wishes. Those wishes should generally include broiled or grilled fish or fowl, as dry as possible; no gravy; no butter on vegetables; salad dressings on the side; and controlled portions. Most restauranteurs want to accommodate their patrons. In a 1993 survey conducted by MasterCard, more than 90 percent of the restauranteurs who were surveyed said they preferred hearing complaints about orders directly. They want you to be satisfied and to bring your business back to them. Still, some servers resist providing you with the information you want about food preparation. Remind yourself of your right to the information, then try making a polite request, even repeated requests if necessary. This strategy should work well most of the time. For example:

Patron: "I'll take the chicken dish with broccoli and new potatoes. How is that prepared?"

Server: "How is what prepared?"

Patron: "The chicken."

Server: "I think it's broiled."

Patron: "In other words, it might be sauteed instead of broiled?"

Server: "Yeah."

Patron: "Could you check on that for me, please?"

Server: "Okay."

(Server leaves for two minutes to check on preparation of the chicken and then returns.)

Server: "It's broiled."

Patron: "Great. Then I'll go with the chicken. I'd like the vegetables grilled, with no butter added on them."

Server: "I don't think they put any butter on the vegetables or the potatoes."

*Patron:* "Please be sure that no butter or any sauces are added to the broccoli or the potatoes, okay?"

*Server:* "Okay."

Does this patron seem overly pushy to you? If you answered yes, you still have a problem. It is critical for you to accept and learn to live by your personal right to get what you pay for. That includes knowing what you're getting. You have a right to know how your food is prepared and to have it prepared according to your wishes. If your server does not comply with reasonable requests for this kind of information, you can ask to speak to the manager or the owner of the restaurant. You could also leave the restaurant. What does not work is to stay and eat foods that contain components that you want to avoid. Why would you pay for something that you are unwilling to eat under most circumstances?

### Eating Out in Ethnic Restaurants: Good Food Choices

The following are some examples of ethnic restaurants with good food choices for each type of cuisine. Each type of cuisine includes some specific Chicago restaurants of that type with information about the calories in specific dishes from those restaurants. This latter information was compiled by nutritionists in a useful book entitled *Dining Lite Chicago*, by Victoria and Valerie Nager. Examples from Chicago are presented to give you an idea of the specific types of healthful meals that you can find.

**Cajun:** Seafood or vegetable gumbo or jumbalaya, grilled fish

- Benedict's blackened yellow fin tuna, 410 calories
- Chicago Bar and Grill's grilled cajun shrimp, 350 calories
- Cuban Village's lobster creole Ackerman, 284 calories

**Chinese:** Stir-fried chicken, seafood, and vegetables; soups (hot and sour, chicken, vegetable); chicken and shrimp dishes steamed without sauces

- Imperial Cathay's Canton lobster, 485 calories; steamed fish, 546 calories
- Memories of China's chicken with vegetables, 409 calories; sauteed pike with broccoli, 362 calories

**French:** Poached, grilled, or steamed fish; chicken and wine sauce; Nicoise salads

- Cafe Bernard's halibut, grilled with tomatoes and capers, 275 calories; swordfish, broiled with citrus, 435 calories; scrod sautee with almonds, 315 calories; broiled chicken with rosemary, 392 calories

- The Everest Room's Maine sea scallop salad, 305 calories; filet of turbot with carrots and leek sauce, 340 calories

**Greek:** Chicken shish kebab; salads, couscous, tabouli

- Greek Islands' broiled swordfish shish kebab (without sauce), 350 calories; Lake Superior whitefish (ask for low-oil preparation), 440 calories; Horta Vasta (large portion dandelion greens—requested without oil), 53 calories
- Dianna's Opaa's broiled chicken, 401 calories; broiled red snapper, 352 calories

**Indian:** Tandoori chicken, vegetable curry, fish

- Bukhara's tiger prawns, 335 calories; tandoori Murgh (tandoori barbecued chicken), 513 calories; Shimla Mirch tandoori (stuffed, spiced bell peppers), 234 calories

**Italian:** Pasta with red clam sauce, meatless marinara, pesto or mushroom sauce (without cream); pizza with no cheese, and fresh vegetable toppings; minestrone soup

- Leona's minestrone soup, 105 calories
- Carlucci's Capelli v'an di pomodoro (angel hair pasta with tomato), 357 calories; linguine ai Gamberi (half portion linguine with shrimp), 327 calories

**Japanese:** Sushi, chicken and fish teriyaki, tofu, and vegetables

- Benihana's hibachi shrimp, 384 calories; hibachi chicken, 400 calories
- Honda's sashimi teishoku (assortment of raw seafood and Japanese horseradish), 139 calories; California roll (avocado and crab sushi, rolled in rice and seaweed), 35 calories

**Mexican:** Chicken and seafood enchiladas with no cheese; tamales with no cheese; chicken or shrimp fajitas (without sour cream); chicken taco salad

- Baja Beach Club's peel your own shrimp (1 lb.), 285 calories; chicken fajitas (does not include guacamole, rice, or beans), 463 calories

- Fernando's chalupa compwesta (beef and chicken tostadas—does not include cheese), 527 calories; ensalada de pollo (chicken salad), 319 calories

**Thai:** Soups, especially sweet and sour soup, chicken salads, stir-fried shrimp and chicken dishes

- Star of Siam's Tom Yum soup (sweet and sour), 131 calories; Yum Woon Sen (silver bean thread salad), 218 calories; Naem Sond (chicken salad), 414 calories; curry chicken special on rice, 536 calories; fried spicy basil leaves with shrimp, 256 calories; Pad Prik (hot and spicy shrimp), 271 calories
- Royal Thai Orchard's royal vegetables with chicken, 406 calories; Pad Kra Praw with chicken, 348 calories

# Key Principles

- Our hunter-gatherer bodies have not as yet adapted to the luxury of modern sedentary lifestyles.

- To lose weight, you must achieve a "negative energy balance" (taking in less energy than your body expends).

- The amount or intensity of hunger (defined here as the desire for food) is affected by biology, emotions, time of day, usual routines, sugar and protein consumption, presence of foods (particularly highly appealing and attractive foods), talking about food, thinking about food, eating by others, drinking alcohol and use of other recreational drugs, exercise and lack of exercise, negative thoughts, variety/blandness of diet, and stimuli that are associated with eating. Hunger is much more complex than most people think.

- Six classes of nutrients (components of food that provide essential elements needed by the body) are (1) carbohydrates (starches, sugars, and fiber); (2) proteins (22 amino acids); (3) fats (saturated, monounsaturated, and polyunsaturated fatty acids); (4) minerals (macronutrients, micronutrients); (5) vitamins (fat soluble, water soluble); (6) water.

- The U.S. Department of Agriculture advocates using the food guide pyramid to provide a balanced diet. The pyramid includes 6 to 11 servings from the grain group (the foundation to the pyramid), 2 to 4 servings from the fruit group, 3 to 5 servings from the vegetable group, 2 to 3 servings from the milk group, and 2 to 3 servings from the meat group.

- The National Cancer Institute recommends that Americans eat 20 to 35 grams of fiber per day (approximately twice the amount that Americans currently consume). Fiber is the undigestible part of plants. Fiber-rich foods include whole grains, fruits, and vegetables.

- There are many benefits to drinking eight 8-ounce glasses of noncaffeinated fluids every day, plus an additional glass for every 25 pounds of excess weight.

- Foods that are high in fat create special problems for weight controllers: fats beget fat. If you can keep 10 to 20 percent of your total calories per day consumed as fat, then you will find it much easier to lose weight and maintain weight losses.

- Some helpful ideas for maintaining a low-fat eating plan include using air-popped popcorn, pretzels, fruit, rice cakes, and raw vegetables for snacks; using mustard, salsa, and spicy peppers to flavor everything; using stir-fried cooking techniques and grilling whenever possible.

- From the standpoint of losing weight, a fat is a fat is a fat. All fats contain similar numbers of calories and similar problems for people who are trying to control their weight.

- Cholesterol is a waxy, fat-like substance found in all animal products. Excess cholesterol can block your arteries, resulting in damage to various organs, including the heart and brain. It is important to know your total cholesterol, LDL cholesterol, and HDL cholesterol levels and to compare them to the recommended standards. The best method of lowering cholesterol levels is to lose weight and to cut down on sources of cholesterol in your food intake. But remember, cholesterol levels do not affect weight control. To lose weight, it is critical to use a low-fat eating plan. Low-fat eating can also improve cholesterol levels.

- Sugar begets more sugar. It is most helpful to avoid eating any sugary snacks, sugary breakfast cereals, and all desserts other than fruit.

- Traveling produces many frustrations, little control, and surrounds you with temptations. To cope when traveling by plane, bring low-fat snacks with you; use traveling as an opportunity to seek out activity and avoid snacking; plan and monitor as obsessively as possible.

- To avoid pitfalls during holidays, plan ahead; avoid starvation before celebration; scope out the food scene at parties; use a food plan; and refocus your holiday season on special people, projects, and finding creative ways to relax.

- When eating in restaurants, remember that you have the right to get what you pay for. This includes having the food you order prepared in accord with your wishes. Healthful alternatives are now readily available at virtually all restaurants.

# Epilogue

## The World's Most Famous Order of Wheat Toast

"I'd like some wheat toast, please," said Jack Nicholson's Bob Dupea in the movie *Five Easy Pieces*.

"Sir, you can only order what's on the menu," responded the waitress in the roadside diner.

"I don't understand. Do you have wheat bread?" replied Bob Dupea.

"Yeah." responded the waitress.

"Do you have a toaster?" asked Dupea.

"Yeah," answered the waitress.

"Then, why can't you put the wheat bread in the toaster and make wheat toast?" inquired Dupea.

"Like I said before, you can only order what's on the menu," the waitress answered rather sternly.

"Okay, I'll make it as easy for you as I can. I'd like ... a chicken salad sandwich on wheat toast. No mayonnaise, no butter, no lettuce," said Dupea.

"A number two," the waitress called out. "Chicken sal san. Hold the butter, the lettuce, and the mayo. . . . Anything else?"

"Yeah," he answered.

"Now all you have to do is hold the chicken, bring me the toast, give me a check for the chicken salad sandwich, and you haven't broken any rules!"

# 5

# Eating Plans

The following excerpt is from the first popular book on dieting, *Letter on Corpulence, Addressed to the Public,* by William Banting (published in Kensington, England, in December 1863).

> Of all the parasites that affect humanity I do not know of, nor can I imagine, any more distressing than that of obesity, and, having just emerged from a very long probation in this affliction, I am desirous of circulating my humble knowledge and experience for the benefit of my fellow man, with an earnest hope it may lead to the same comfort and happiness I now feel under the extraordinary change— which might almost be termed miraculous had it not been accomplished by the most simple common-sense means.
>
> For the sake of argument and illustration I will presume that certain articles of ordinary diet, however beneficial in youth, are prejudicial in advanced life, like beans to a horse, whose common ordinary food is hay and corn. It may be useful food occasionally, under peculiar circumstances, but detrimental as a constancy. I will, therefore, adopt the analogy, and call such food human beans. The items from which I was advised (by my physician, Dr. William Harvey) to abstain as much as possible were: bread, butter, milk, sugar, beer, and potatoes, which had been the main (and I thought innocent) elements of my existence, or at all events they had for many years been adopted freely.
>
> These, said my excellent adviser, contain starch and saccharine matter, tending to create fat, and should be avoided altogether. At the first blush it seemed to me that I had little left to live upon, but my kind friend soon showed

me there was ample, and I was only too happy to give the plan a fair trial, and, within a very few days, found immense benefit from it. It may better elucidate the dietary plan if I describe generally what I have sanction to take, and that man must be an extraordinary person who would desire a better table:—

For breakfast, I take four or five ounces of beef, muton [sic], kidneys, broiled fish, bacon, or cold meat of any kind except pork; a large cup of tea (without milk or sugar), a little biscuit, or one ounce of dry toast.

For dinner, five or six ounces of any fish except salmon, any meat except pork, any vegetable except potato, one ounce of dry toast, fruit out of a pudding, any kind of poultry or game, and two or three glasses of good claret, sherry, or Madeira-Champagne, Port and Beer forbidden.

For tea, two or three ounces of fruit, a rusk or two, and a cup of tea without milk or sugar.

For supper, three or four ounces of meat or fish, similar to dinner, with a glass or two of claret.

For nightcap, if required, a tumbler of grog—(gin, whisky, or brandy, without sugar)—or a glass or two of claret or sherry.

This plan leads to an excellent night's rest, with from six to eight hours' sound sleep. The dry toast or rusk may have a tablespoonful of spirit to soften it, which will prove acceptable. Perhaps I did not wholly escape starchy or saccharine matter, but scrupulously avoided those beans, such as milk, sugar, beer, butter & c.[sic], which were known to contain them.

Experience has taught me to believe that these human beans are the most insidious enemies man, with a tendency to corpulence in advanced life, can possess, though eminently friendly to youth. He may very prudently mount guard against such an enemy if he is not a fool to himself, and I fervently hope this truthful unvarnished tale may lead him to make a trial of my plan, which I sincerely recommend to public notice,—not with any ambitious motive, but in sincere good faith to help my fellow-creatures to obtain the marvelous blessings I have found within the short period of a few months.

I have not felt so well as now for the last twenty years.

Have suffered no inconvenience whatever in the probational remedy.

Am reduced many inches in bulk, and 35 lbs. in weight in thirty-eight weeks.

Come down stairs forward naturally, with perfect ease.

Go up stairs and take ordinary exercise freely, without the slightest inconvenience.

Can perform every necessary office for myself.

The umbilical rupture is greatly ameliorated, and gives me no anxiety.

My sight is restored—my hearing improved.

My other bodily ailments are ameliorated; indeed, almost past into matter of history.

William Banting sought only to relieve "suffering humanity" by distributing the dietary plan to which he attributed his successful weight reduction. His booklet on the subject was reprinted ten times during the first 40 years after its initial publication. More than 100,000 copies of it were distributed for free or sold. It met with great enthusiasm and tremendous controversy, as well. Many people expressed outrage about even discussing obesity and weight control. For example, an editorial appearing in the January 25, 1865 issue of *Commercial Advertiser* exclaimed:

Good heavens! The ill of the world is not repletion, it is emptiness and all the other fat men are running about in their own puffery and breathless manner asking: What about malt? How is it as to chocolate? Are anchovies bad for me? Must I cut off my stilton? To these I say: Let me be your doctor. Retrench your all-absorbing self interest. Turn your thoughts from your duodenum to the famishing creatures who peer down through the railings of your areas at the blazing fire in your kitchen grate. Give up this filthy selfishness that takes for its worship all that is least worthy in humanity. Walk, ride, bath, swim, fast if you must, but take your thoughts off this detestable theme and try to remember that the subject you want to popularize is in its details one of the coarsest that can be made matter for conversation.

William Banting's motives were pure, but his "Banting System" created a great moral controversy. The dietary plan he recommended was based on some notions from the midnineteenth century about the manner in which the liver works. The actual dietary plan emphasized protein intake in accord with these views. The Banting System recommends consuming more than twice as much protein as the current dietary recommendations endorsed by the U.S. Department of Agriculture. Many subsequent best sellers also emphasize high protein diets. Very few current dietary plans, however, suggest consuming 23 percent of one's calories in alcohol! The Banting System did this. Quite a remarkable recommendation, by today's standards of health.

# Diets Don't Work

The Banting System appears quaint by 1994 standards. People no longer talk about "taking" their meals or desiring "a better table." Yet they buy millions of books and magazines offering new dietary plans every year. Does the Banting System work? Do any diets work? One best seller made its reputation by asserting, "Diets don't work!" This simple statement is true. Diets provide too much structure, too few options, and too many limitations for almost anyone to live with for very long. It doesn't matter what the diet is. Very few people can restrict their eating to relatively narrow ranges of foods for very long. You go to parties, to dinners at friends' houses, and you face too many types of foods to say no to every-thing but the 10, 12, 15, or even 50 foods that are part of any one diet. The Banting System was widely read and attempted in the nineteenth century. In fact, the term "Banting System" became synonymous with di-eting for several decades. But you probably never heard of it until reading these passages, right? All that means is that diet crazes come and go. Some last a few weeks, while others last many years, but they all disap-pear eventually.

This chapter includes five structured eating plans, despite the fact that people do not stick with any one dietary plan for very long. I have found during the last 20 years that many people like to use structured eating plans occasionally. In other words, sometimes weight controllers try different eating plans in order to break problematic habits. Some peo-ple swear off sugar for a while. Others adopt the latest best-selling diet plan. Many people try the relatively unstructured, and very reasonable, dietary plan offered by Weight Watchers. For these reasons, this chapter offers the following eating plans and some ideas about how to use them to focus your attention on persistence.

- Self-Monitoring plan
- "Almost Never" plan
- Popcorn plan
- Vegetarian plan
- Very low-calorie diet (VLCD)

# The Self-Monitoring Plan: Dieting Without a Diet

Most experts on the treatment of obesity agree on at least one thing: Self-monitoring is the single most important element of effective weight con-trol. Self-monitoring is the systematic or careful observation and recording of behavior that you wish to change. For weight controllers, self-monitoring involves observing and recording eating and exercising behaviors. For example, the following form is one that my clients have used for many years:

---

# Self-Monitoring Diary

Date: _____

*Exercise:*

_____

| Time | Food | Calories | Fat |
|------|------|----------|-----|
|      |      |          |     |

Total Cals./Fat gms:  _____     _____

---

If you could get yourself to write down everything you eat and all of your exercising for the next ten years, you would *certainly* become an effective weight controller. This is a very dramatic statement. It means that what you eat is less important than your ability to observe and record your eating and exercising. If you could get yourself to observe, record, and think about your eating and exercising every single day, you would modify your eating and exercising behaviors to keep yourself healthier. There are many complicated explanations for this. The simple version is: People are goal-oriented creatures. If you have clear goals in mind, you attempt to reach them. The main challenge is to stay aware of yourself in pursuit of that goal. If you maintain a consistent awareness, you will strive to reach that goal. This isn't true for everybody all of the time. But these principles hold for most people, most of the time.

## Effects of Consistent Self-Monitoring

Some dramatic examples from research on weight control illustrate the power of self-monitoring. In 1982, E. B. Fisher, Michael Lowe, and their colleagues found that weight controllers who discontinued self-monitoring during a three-week holiday season gained 57 times as much weight as their counterparts, who sustained self-monitoring during the holidays. In 1986, Randy Flanery and I reported that self-monitoring was the only one out of ten habits we measured that was associated with successful maintenance of weight loss 1 1/2 years after treatment ended. Several other researchers found that almost all of their clients reported relying on self-monitoring to help them control their weight during treatment, but only *successful* weight controllers used self-monitoring regularly one year or more after treatment.

In a study published in 1993, Ray Baker and I provided further evidence about the critical role of self-monitoring in effective weight control. The two graphs shown on the next page indicate that weight controllers who were most consistent in their monitoring (quartile 4) lost substantially more weight than people who were more inconsistent at self-monitoring. The top graph shows that 100 percent of the most consistent self-monitors lost at least some weight at the end of 12 and 18 weeks; less than 40 percent of the least consistent self-monitors lost weight. The bottom graph shows that at the end of 18 weeks (which included the Thanksgiving to New Year's holiday season), participants in our weight control program actually gained, on average, close to 10 pounds if their monitoring was very inconsistent (quartile 1). The most consistent monitors, by contrast, lost an average of 30 pounds during that 18-week period. Consider that result carefully. Inconsistent monitors gained 10, while consistent monitors lost 30.

These research findings emphasize that:

**If you can self-monitor everything you eat, you can control your weight.**

This assertion applies to most people, most of the time. Unfortunately, very unfortunately, most people have great difficulty persisting at self-monitoring. Ninety percent of people involved in weight control programs conducted by professionals can self-monitor while they participate in these programs. Very few people seem able to maintain consistent self-monitoring without a program to support and encourage them to do so. On the other hand, some people can self-monitor effectively even when pursuing effective weight control on their own. Others find that with the support of a low-cost program, such as Weight Watchers, they can get themselves to monitor very consistently and effectively.

## Self-Monitoring Techniques

If you haven't tried self-monitoring on your own, why not try doing so for the next day or week? You can buy a small notebook from any bookstore. Most people like very small notebooks that they put in their pockets or purses. You could simply use the self-monitoring form pre-

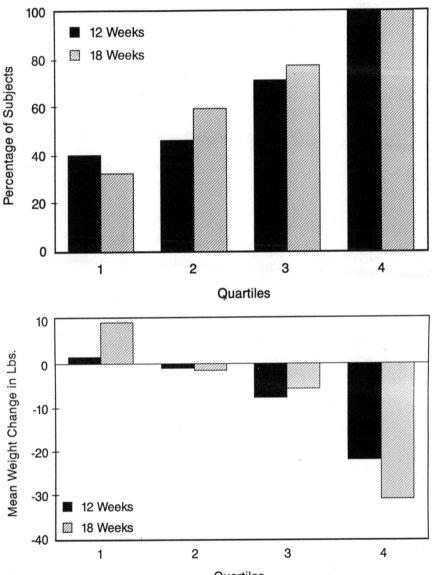

sented earlier, recording the date, time, food consumed and amount, calories consumed, and fat grams consumed. You could also enter the total
number of calories consumed each day and the percentage of those calories coming from fat, using the formulas presented in Chapter 4 (nine
calories per gram of fat). In our research, Ray Baker and I discovered
that the most important thing is not whether you record calories and fat
grams; it is whether you record what you eat very consistently—every
day.

You may find that you are able to sustain self-monitoring without the assistance of any program or other forms of encouragement. If you are one of the few people who can do this consistently, and that means every day, then you have just discovered the most effective "eating plan" you could find. Try spending the one to three minutes per day to write down exactly what you eat; you'll see that if you sustain this effort, you will control your weight.

If you are one of the vast majority of people who cannot sustain self-monitoring on your own, consider joining Weight Watchers or some other inexpensive group or program (such as Take Off Pounds Sensibly, a no-cost club available in most metropolitan areas in the United States). These support groups can help you stay focused enough to sustain your self-monitoring. If that doesn't do the trick for you, consider joining a professionally conducted program for weight control. These programs are almost always directed by psychologists. You may be able to find such a program in your area by calling your local hospital or university. Ask for the psychology department and inquire about a weight control program conducted by a psychologist who specializes in "cognitive-behavior therapy." If this doesn't work, you can identify psychologists in your area who specialize in this approach by calling the Association for Advancement of Behavior Therapy (15 West 36th Street, New York, NY 10018, 212/279-7970).

## The "Almost Never" Plan

"I know what to do, it's getting myself to do it—that's the problem."

I've heard this statement and versions of it hundreds of times. Scientific research also supports it. Studies show that when weight controllers begin a program, regardless of the content of the program, they often make healthful changes in their eating and exercising habits. People have much greater difficulty staying focused and persisting than they do understanding the basic rules of weight control. In other words, weight controllers know that burgers and fries are very problematic, while salads and grilled chicken are fine. Nevertheless, many people don't understand the degree to which certain rules apply. For example, how many people really have a complete understanding of some of the biological forces that make weight control so challenging? Most people do not appreciate the degree to which fat and sugar present major biological challenges. Because of this, I find that it is helpful to state very clearly some rules to live by for effective weight control. These rules include types of food to avoid as much as possible (the "Almost Never" rules) and principles of eating to follow as much as possible (the "Almost Always" rules). Take a look at the list of Almost Never and the Almost Always rules that follow and see what you think.

## Almost Never: Principles for Avoiding Problematic Foods

It would be extremely helpful for effective weight control to eat the following foods and preparations "almost never." Occasional, very rare consumption of these foods and types of food preparations is expected. But *each incident* in which these foods are eaten is best viewed as a problem. It is not sinful, shameful, horrible, or awful to deviate from this plan. These deviations are problems to be solved. Successful weight controllers solve these problems well and "almost never" consume the foods on this list.

Almost never eat:

Fried foods (except "stir fries")

Desserts other than fruit

High-fat lunch meats (bologna, salami)

Candy (candy bars, truffles)

Regular salad dressings (especially those served on the salad, not on the side)

Cookies, brownies, cake

Mayonnaise (except fat-free mayonnaise)

Cheese (other than no-fat or very low-fat cheese, 2 grams of fat per ounce or less

Ice cream and ice cream products (milkshakes, malts)

Gravy and other high-fat sauces

## Almost Always Rules

Almost always eat:

Low-fat, low-sugar foods

Low-fat, low-sugar snacks (popcorn, pretzels, fruit, rice cakes, low-calorie jello, low-calorie cocoa)

Grilled fish and fowl

Vegetables

Salads (dressing on the side, preferably low-calorie and low-fat; use your own if possible)

Mustard on sandwiches

Spicy foods

Salsa on practically everything

Pastas (with tomato sauces, plain)

Weight controllers often ask questions like the following ones after reviewing these "almost always/almost never" principles:

### What about pizza, frozen yogurt, birthday cakes, and sauces?

**Question:** What about pizza? Pizza, after all, has all of the food groups.

**Answer:** Pizzas often contain vegetables, dairy, meat, and grains. They do, indeed, provide a wide range of food groups. This fact would be very important if you were starving on a desert island. However, pizza also contains many calories, and many of those calories come from fat. For example, two slices of a Godfather's Stuffed Pizza Cheese Combo contain 860 calories and 40 grams of fat (42 percent of the calories come from fat). Even Godfather's less caloric pizzas, as well as Pizza Hut's full range of pizza offerings, contain 30 to 50 percent of the calories from fat. Pizza cheese (mozzarella), made with part-skim milk, is *still* a high-fat food. A majority of the calories of virtually all cheeses (aside from the no-fat or very low-fat versions) come from saturated fat. Pizzas often have a lot of cheese on them.

The good news is that many places serve pizzas without any cheese. Pizza without cheese represents a reasonable food choice. The crust in some pizzas contains significant amounts of fat, but as an alternative food, certainly for occasional purposes, pizzas with no cheese can work quite well.

If you are trapped in a meeting and surrounded by pizzas, what can you do? You can perform minor surgery and remove the cheese from your slices of pizza. Some people find this distasteful. Although not the most acceptable form of behavior, it could work a lot better for you than to eat high-fat food and negate your efforts at effective weight control.

**Question:** What about frozen yogurt?

**Answer:** Many frozen yogurts fulfill the low-fat "Almost Always" rule. However, they can be surprisingly high in fat content and, therefore, come close to violating the ice cream "Almost Never" rule. If you are selective and read labels carefully, you can find low-fat frozen yogurts. Remember that most frozen yogurts contain a lot of sweetener. This could trigger some of the same reactions that other sugary foods do.

Many weight controllers use frozen yogurts in modest amounts as a treat, which is a reasonable approach. Just be careful of some establishments that serve nearly twice the amounts that they advertise for a given price. Try ordering the smallest, child-size portion available at a frozen yogurt stand or restaurant. Frozen yogurt can also become problematic if it is purchased in pints, quarts, or larger bulk quantities. Many people find themselves dipping into these treats more often than they would like. So the answer is—use frozen yogurt with caution.

**Question:** What about birthday cake?

**Answer:** Birthday cakes are an important tradition to many people. However, traditions can change. Why would you want to eat a food that creates a problem for you in celebration of a special day? When you first had a birthday cake to celebrate your birthday during childhood, you didn't realize the kind of problem that foods high in sugar and fat create for you. In fact, at that time, you probably didn't have such a problem. Now you have new information that advises against consuming foods like cake. In the 1950s, practically every dinner table in America had red meat on it. That tradition has changed. In William Banting's day (mid-1800s), drinking liberal quantities of alcohol was traditional. That tradition has also changed. It is now time for you to consider changing the birthday cake tradition for yourself. This position seems rather extreme to many people. However, weight control takes extreme focusing and persistence. If you really want to succeed at this difficult challenge, you must take difficult steps.

Another problem with allowing yourself a birthday cake concerns permission. If you give yourself permission for this deviation from the plan, what else will you permit? What about other holidays? What about other people's birthdays? What about your children's birthdays? Some of the clients with whom I've worked give themselves permission to eat problematic foods when they are hungry, tired, on vacation, at someone else's house for dinner or for a party, when they are sad or depressed, . . . . The list goes on and on.

Permissions often create problems. For example, if you give yourself permission to eat problematic food today, then you may struggle mightily with other food decisions tomorrow. These struggles take their toll. Instead of food becoming more secondary in your life, the struggle becomes primary. Lots of struggles can put you into a major frustration stage. This is an unpleasant stage that often produces unfavorable results. In other words, if you use permissions to allow yourself to eat problematic foods, it can lead to excessive struggling with food choices and decreased commitment and persistence. All of these problems from a birthday cake? Perhaps!

**Question:** How can you tell about sauces in restaurants?

**Answer:** You can assume that any sauce made in a restaurant with oil as a primary ingredient is problematic. On the other hand, tomato sauces, marinara sauces, and sauces that are essentially broths (which are available increasingly in restaurants) are quite acceptable. Any sauces made with cheese (such as Alfredo sauce) are very high in fat. Similarly, sauces and soups with cream bases are high-fat foods.

One of my clients recently told a story about a mushroom soup. His dining companion ordered a seemingly innocuous mushroom soup. His companion raved about how wonderful the soup was, and it looked very appealing to the client. When my client tasted the soup, he soon realized that its primary ingredient was butter. The word "mushroom" suggests a low-fat, safe vegetable base. As Americans become increasingly health conscious, restauranteurs and food packagers will market and name products to suggest their healthfulness. You can generally assume the worst: if you're not sure about the ingredients in a product, it would be wise to avoid it. In a restaurant, try to order only items for which you know the fat and sugar contents. These guidelines sound stringent. Unfortunately, your biology demands such stringencies. Successful weight controllers follow these guidelines with tremendous consistency.

Most diets provide numerous recipes. Because recipes are often detailed and sometimes hard to follow, people do not use them very much. The central ideas in the recipes can, however, provide helpful guidance about low-fat and low-sugar meals. Breakfast and lunch seem less challenging for most weight controllers than dinner. No-fat cereals that have no sugar or very little sugar mixed with skim milk, and bagels or low-calorie bread and no-fat cheese are simple and effective breakfasts. Common lunches include turkey or chicken sandwiches, salads with low-fat dressing, broth-based soups, and fruit. In the United States, dinners and the evening more generally present the biggest challenge for weight controllers. People relax more in the evening, decrease their focus on goals, and eat in a more elaborate and leisurely manner than they do during the day. My clients use the ideas presented in the following list to help them follow the principles of the "Almost Never" plan during this most challenging time of the day. You will notice that the list focuses on central ideas about meals rather than presenting highly specific formulas for how to prepare them. You might find this approach more useful than the usual method of presenting recipes. If you take the ideas and experiment with them to make them your own, you will build your own set of mainstay meals for dinner based on the "Almost Never" plan.

## Favorite Dinner Ideas From the "Almost Never" Plan

**Healthy Choice lean ground beef.** This is a beef and grain combination, available in frozen food sections), with 28 percent of calories from fat, and 56 percent fewer calories than lean ground beef. Use it to make tacos and chili:

- Tacos: Combine (for one serving) four ounces of Healthy Choice lean ground beef with Tio Sanchez or some other taco seasoning packet in a frying pan (no need to add oil). Add canned tomatoes if desired. After cooking, add fresh chopped vegetables (for example, bell peppers, lettuce, cucumbers, tomatoes) and salsa. Serve over Spanish rice or serve in flour or corn tortilla shells.

- Chili: Combine with light red kidney beans, canned tomatoes, chili, onion powder, and garlic. Use 8 or 16 ounces of Healthy Choice lean ground beef and freeze leftovers. Serve over macaroni.

**Pasta.** Combine any type of pasta with low-fat, low-calorie tomato sauces (for example, Healthy Choice, Ragu "Today's Recipe," Ci Bella.) They should have 40 to 50 calories for one-half cup. Combine with one whole or one-half can of clams and use salsa if desired.

**Baked potatoes.** Bake in microwave and combine with no-fat or 1 percent cottage cheese or plain yogurt and broccoli and salsa, if desired. Or consider melting no-fat mozzarella cheese on top of a baked potato.

**Grilled vegetables.** Lightly coat any vegetables (for example, carrots, peppers, zucchini, onions, potatoes) with olive oil and broil with garlic. Cook a large quantity and eat with no-fat or low-fat yogurt.

**Stir-fries.** Use cilantro, garlic, parsley, and experiment with a variety of other species to create seasonings (for example, consider using dried red peppers and sliced ginger to create particularly spicy dishes). Stir-fry in water or use Pam or other no-fat cooking agent. Combine with frozen, peeled shrimp and an assortment of vegetables. Serve over rice. Turkey breast or chicken breast without skin can be substituted for the shrimp. It helps to get a wok with a Teflon or other non-stick cooking surface.

**Frozen entrees and low-fat soups.** Check ingredients carefully and combine these mini-meals with fresh salads and fruit. (Healthy Choice soups and a wide variety of frozen dinners work rather well. In addition, many other soups satisfy the "Almost Never" plan very nicely.

# The Popcorn Plan

The Popcorn plan may help people structure what they eat and limit their eating to safe, yet restricted, amounts. My clients have used a version of this plan for ten years. Many of them say that it provides a useful direction for constructing their own eating plans.

The Popcorn plan gets its name from a central recommendation within it. This plan encourages people to use popcorn (preferably air-popped) as an evening snack. Popcorn provides a tasty treat, dietary fiber (3.1 grams for 3 cups) at a cost of relatively few calories and a small amount of fat. For example, three cups of air-popped popcorn contain 75 calories and approximately 2 grams of fat.

Three cups of popcorn is one of the selections in the following list of "Breads and Starches." This plan includes seven selections of "Proteins," five selections of "Breads and Starches," two "Fruits," and unlimited "Free Vegetables." There are also some foods, listed under a "Miscellaneous" heading, that you can consume as desired, with some exceptions. The following table summarizes the plan.

| Group | Servings per Day |
| --- | --- |
| Proteins | 7 |
| Breads and Starches | 5 |
| Fruits | 2 |
| Free Vegetables | As much as desired |
| Miscellaneous | As much as desired (with some exceptions as noted) |

Food selections are listed on the following pages. You will see that quite a wide variety of foods are available on this plan. However, all foods are to be prepared without any butter or oils. Food preparation is limited to steaming, broiling, grilling, no-fat stir frying, and other methods that add no extra calories.

Several supplements (vitamins, calcium, and potassium) are suggested to ensure your safety. These supplemental requirements are presented following the lists of primary food groups.

The Popcorn plan provides approximately 1000 calories per day. It encourages a style of eating that provides very modest amounts of fat (less than 20 percent of total calories consumed). Four sample menus follow the lists of food groups and supplements.

Like all structured eating plans or diets, most people find it difficult to stay within the boundaries of this plan. However, many of my clients have used this plan as a skeleton around which they have constructed their own style of eating. That approach makes sense. There is no value to beating yourself up for not following relatively arbitrary rules. For example, would it really matter if you had six proteins instead of seven combined with six breads and starches instead of five? The answer is no. Perhaps the Popcorn plan can help you develop your own approach. The key to making this work is to provide yourself some leeway. In other words, it may help you to have a structure, but it will certainly hurt you if you become very critical and unforgiving about a normal amount of deviation from that structure.

## Popcorn Plan

**Proteins (7 per day)**
**1 serving = 1 ounce; approximately 50 calories**

Chicken breast without skin          1 oz.
  and trimmed of fat

| | |
|---|---|
| Cheese (no-fat) | 1 oz. |
| Cottage cheese (1% fat) | 1/4 cup = 1 serving |
| Egg whites | 2 = 1 serving, cook with Pam |
| Fish (including shellfish), any kind (for example, tuna, swordfish, clams, shrimp, lobster, catfish, scallops, cod, flounder) | 1 oz. |
| Skim milk | 3/4 cup = 1 serving |
| Turkey breast without skin | 1 oz. |
| Veal, dark meat of chicken | Limit to 2 servings per week |

### Breads and Starches (5 per day)
### 1 serving = 1 selection; approximately 80 calories

*Breads*

| | |
|---|---|
| Bagel | 1/2 small |
| Bialy | 1 |
| White (also French and Italian) | 1 slice |
| Whole wheat | 1 slice |
| Rye/pumpernickel | 1 slice |
| Raisin (no icing) | 1 slice |
| Bread crumbs, dry | 3 Tbsp |
| Bread sticks (7 in. long x 3/4 in. diameter) | 4 |
| Bun, hamburger or hot dog | 1/2 |
| Croutons, plain | 1/2 cup |
| English muffin | 1/2 small |
| Melba toast, oblong | 4 |
| Melba toast, round | 8 |
| Pita (8 in. diameter) | 1/2 |
| Rolls, pan or hard | 1/2 large, 1 small |
| Rusk | 2 |
| Tortilla, corn or flour (6 in. diameter) | 1 |

*Cereals*

| | |
|---|---|
| Cooked | 1/2 cup |
| Grits | 1/2 cup |

| | |
|---|---|
| Ready-to-eat, dry and no sugar coating | 3/4 cup |
| Bran, all types but check calories | 1/3 to 2/3 cup |
| GrapeNuts | 3 Tbsp |
| Puffed wheat/puffed rice | 1 cup |
| Shredded wheat biscuits | 1 large or 1/2 cup spoon size |

*Starchy Vegetables*

| | |
|---|---|
| Baked beans, no pork | 1/4 cup |
| Corn, whole kernel | 1/3 cup |
| Corn, ear (4 in. long) | 1 |
| Popcorn (air-popped) | 3 cups |
| Dried beans and peas, cooked | 1/2 cup |
| Lentils | 1/2 cup |
| Lima beans | 1/2 cup |
| Mixed vegetables | 1/2 cup |
| Parsnips | 2/3 cup |
| Peas, green | 1/2 cup |
| Potato, white | 1 small, 1/2 cup mashed |
| Potato, sweet or yams | 1/4 cup |
| Pumpkin | 3/4 cup |
| Squash: acorn, hubbard, butternut | 1/2 cup |

*Note: I recommend that you have popcorn for one of your selections every day.*

*Crackers*

| | |
|---|---|
| Matzo (6 in. square) | 1 |
| Oyster | 20 or 1/2 cup |
| Rye wafers (2 in. x 3 1/2 in.) | 3 |
| Saltines | 6 |
| Soda (2 1/2 in. square) | 4 |
| Zwieback | 2 |

*Pastas and Grains*

| | |
|---|---|
| Barley, pearl, dry | 1 1/2 Tbsp |
| Macaroni, cooked | 1/2 cup |

| Noodles, cooked | 1/2 cup |
| Rice, cooked | 1/2 cup |
| Spaghetti/other pasta, cooked | 1/2 cup |
| Wheat germ | 1/4 cup |

### Fruits (2 per day)
### 1 serving = 80 calories, approx.

Any type. The most desirable (for potassium needs) are grapefruit, banana, cantaloupe, and nectarine.

### Free vegetables
### Raw or steamed as desired

| | |
|---|---|
| Alfalfa sprouts | Broccoli |
| Cabbage | Cauliflower |
| Celery | Chicory |
| Chinese Cabbage | Chives |
| Cucumbers | Endive |
| Escarole | Lettuce |
| Mushrooms | Parsley |
| Peppers | Radishes |
| Tomatoes (1/2 cup) | Spinach |
| Zucchini | Watercress |

### Miscellaneous
### Use/eat as desired unless otherwise noted

*Baking Aids*

| | |
|---|---|
| Baking powder | Baking soda |
| Cream of tartar | Flavoring extracts, pure |
| Yeast, baking | |

*Beverages*

| | |
|---|---|
| Clam juice (limit to 1/2 cup per day) | Club soda |
| Coffee | Decaffeinated coffee |
| Decaffeinated tea | Carbonated water |
| Mineral water | Postum (limit to 1 tsp per meal) |
| Sugar-free carbonated drinks | Sauerkraut juice (limit to 1 cup per day) |

*Condiments*

Artificial sweetener

Hot pepper sauce

Mustard, prepared

Pimento

Tabasco sauce

Vinegar

Herbed vinegar

Horseradish

Pickles, unsweetened

Salsa

Taco sauce

Worcestershire sauce

*Soups*

Beef tea

Broth, without fat

Bouillon cubes, prepared with
water

*Seasonings*

Herbs (for example, sage,
oregano, thyme, basil)

Garlic, garlic powder, garlic
salt, garlic juice

Mustard, dry

Pepper

Poppy seed

Salt, seasoned salt, salt
substitutes

Tenderizers

Celery seed or celery salt

Mint leaves

Onion salt, onion powder, onion
flakes, onion juice

Paprika

Poultry seasoning

Spices (for example, cloves,
cinnamon, ginger, cumin)

*Limit to 2 Tbsp per day*

Chili sauce, without sugar

Cocktail sauce

Salad dressings—only those
with 20 calories or less per
Tbsp (no-fat, preferred)

Yeast, brewers

Jam and jelly, artificially
sweetened

Cocoa, dry unsweetened powder

Soy sauce

**Required Supplements**

One multivitamin per day

600 mg calcium per day

16 mEq potassium chloride per
day (may require prescription
for Slow K or Micro K)

*Other*

Cranberries, unsweetened

Lime (limit to 2 per day or 1/4 cup juice per day)

Lemon (limit to 1 per day or 1/4 cup juice per day)

Gelatin, unflavored or artificially sweetened

Here are four sample menus that follow the Popcorn plan:

## Sample Menu #1

| | |
|---|---|
| **Breakfast** | 1/2 bagel (or 1 bialy) |
| | 2 oz. lox |
| **Snack** | Celery sticks and cucumber slices |
| **Lunch** | 2 oz. tuna with Mrs. Pickford's no oil salad dressing |
| | 3/4 cup skim milk |
| | Salad: lettuce, cucumber, green pepper, tomatoes with vinegar, lemon juice, or 1 Tbsp of no-oil dressing |
| | 1/2 slice rye toast |
| **Snack** | Radishes, zucchini slices, 1 apple |
| **Dinner** | 3 oz. bass with lemon juice, parsley flakes, and garlic powder |
| | 1 medium baked potato |
| | Salad: sliced fresh mushrooms on a bed of raw fresh spinach, sprinkled with herbed vinegar or lemon juice |
| | 3/4 cup skim milk |
| | 1 orange |
| **Snack** | 3 cups air-popped popcorn |

## Sample Menu #2

| | |
|---|---|
| **Breakfast** | 3 egg white omelet + 1/2 cup cottage cheese (1% fat) with onion and green pepper |
| | 1 slice cracked wheat bread |
| | 1 grapefruit |
| **Snack** | Celery sticks |
| **Lunch** | 1 cup broth or bouillon (chicken, beef, or vegetable) |

|  | 2 oz. shrimp + 1 oz. turkey breast on romaine lettuce with alfalfa sprouts, green pepper, tomato, celery, and 1 Tbsp of no-oil dressing |
|  | 1 slice cracked wheat bread |
| **Snack** | Cucumber slices, 1 apple |
| **Dinner** | 3 oz. broiled whitefish or swordfish with lemon, rosemary, sage, and thyme |
|  | 1 cup rice |
|  | Salad: raw cabbage with 1 Tbsp of no-oil dressing, vinegar, or lemon juice + celery salt, onion salt or powder, and/or dill |
| **Snack** | 3 cups of air-popped popcorn |

## Sample Menu #3

| **Breakfast** | 1/2 English muffin with 1/4 cup of cottage cheese (1%) and cinnamon, broiled |
|  | 1 banana |
| **Snack** | 1 oz. turkey |
|  | Lettuce leaves |
| **Lunch** | 1 cup broth |
|  | 3 oz. veal sauteed (Pam) with lemon juice, garlic, and basil |
| **Snack** | Green pepper slices, 1 apple |
| **Dinner** | 3 oz. broiled scallops with lemon |
|  | 1/2 cup peas |
|  | Salad: spinach, alfalfa sprouts, and raw zucchini with 1 Tbsp no-oil dressing |
|  | 1 slice Italian bread |
|  | 3/4 cup skim milk |
| **Snack** | 3 cups of air-popped popcorn |

## Sample Menu #4

| **Breakfast** | 2/3 cup bran cereal, with 1 banana sliced on it |
|  | 3/4 cup skim milk |
| **Snack** | Raw mushrooms and celery sticks |
| **Lunch** | 4 oz. chicken breast with hot sauce and grated lettuce |
|  | 1/2 pita bread |

| | |
|---|---|
| **Snack** | Green pepper slices, 1/2 cantaloupe |
| | 1 cup broth or bouillon |
| **Dinner** | 4 oz. broiled snapper with lemon juice and paprika |
| | Salad: lettuce, tomato (1/2 cup) with 1 Tbsp of no-oil dressing |
| **Snack** | 3 cups air-popped popcorn |

## The Vegetarian Plan

If you are a Sylvester Stallone fan, you probably remember Rocky Balboa's power breakfast in the movie *Rocky*: five raw eggs cracked into a glass and swallowed whole. Rocky slurped down that gloppy mixture, supposedly to give himself the extra strength he needed to win his championship fights. He slurped down the eggs and then groggily began his morning run into the streets of Philadelphia. This was the late 1970s' version of the Banting System.

As Mr. Banting advocated a century and a third ago, most Americans still consume about twice as much protein as they need. Most of the proteins consumed come from animal products. In fact, two-thirds of the protein in the average American diet comes from animal products, whereas approximately half of the protein in the American diet at the turn of the century came from animal products. Some animal products contain a lot of protein and very little fat or no fat. For example, one cup of skim milk contains eight grams of protein and no grams of fat (86 calories). In contrast, one cup of whole milk contains the same amount of protein (eight grams), but it also contains eight grams of fat and nearly twice the amount of calories as skim milk. Unfortunately, Americans typically get their protein from higher fat foods.

For weight controllers, fat is of much greater concern than protein. Therein lies the beauty of a vegetarian approach. Vegetarians often consume much of their protein from plant products. Some surveys of the amount of proteins consumed by American vegetarians show that these individuals have no difficulty getting adequate amounts of protein.

The three types of vegetarian diets are:

**Strict or pure vegetarian diet:** Excludes all food of animal origin, including meat, poultry, fish, eggs, and dairy products

**Lacto-ovo vegetarian diet:** Excludes meat, poultry, and fish; includes eggs and dairy products

**Lacto-vegetarian diet:** Excludes meat, poultry, fish, and eggs; includes dairy products

The challenge for all vegetarians is to ensure an adequate supply of protein in the daily diet. Many foods contain proteins, but most plant foods contain "incomplete proteins." Foods with incomplete proteins are deficient in one or more of the nine essential amino acids (components of protein). For example, grains, seeds, and nuts are high in the amino acid methionine, but low in the amino acid lysine. Legumes (dried peas and beans, such as lentils, black-eyed peas, soybeans, chickpeas, kidney beans, pinto beans, and black beans) are high in the amino acid lysine, but low in the amino acid methionine. Fortunately, when you eat complementary sources of amino acids, you get the equivalent of a complete protein. So red beans and rice, peanut butter and jelly sandwiches, tossed salads with almonds, lentil soup with sunflower seeds, and a whole host of other combinations of foods provide complete proteins. *It is not necessary to eat complementary proteins at one meal.* If you had bean soup for lunch and a rice or whole grain pasta salad for dinner, you would provide your body with complete protein. In fact, only strict vegetarians need to be concerned about the adequacy of their diets. *Lacto-ovo and lacto-vegetarian diets will almost undoubtedly provide adequate amounts of complete proteins during the course of the day.*

## Lacto-Ovo Vegetarian

Some people who adopt a lacto-ovo vegetarian diet (the one I recommend the most to people who want to try such an approach) remain concerned about their protein intake. Let's consider this issue in a bit more detail to reassure you about the adequacy of this plan. First, if you're an adult and not pregnant, compute the number of grams in your recommended dietary allowance for protein by multiplying your weight (in pounds) by .36. If you weigh 150 pounds, this calculation suggests that you should consume 54 grams of protein per day. Children, pregnant, and lactating women need more protein than others. For example, infants up to six months of age require an amount of protein in grams equal to their weight every day. For boys and girls 11 through 14, multiply body weight by .45. Pregnant and breast-feeding women are encouraged to consume an extra 10 to 15 grams of protein per day. Similarly, very athletic individuals (including professional athletes) could use an extra 30 or more grams of protein per day. However, since most Americans get more than twice as much as the minimal recommended levels, very few people need to be concerned about the amount of protein that they are consuming.

It is helpful to remember that an ounce of most animal foods contains about seven grams of protein, while plant foods contain much less. Some specific examples are:

| Food | Protein (grams) |
| --- | --- |
| 1 oz. meat, poultry, fish | 7 |
| 1 oz. cheese | 7 |

| | |
|---|---|
| 1 egg | 7 |
| 1 cup milk/yogurt | 8 |
| 1/2 cup vanilla ice cream | 2 |
| 1/2 cup beans | 6 |
| 1 Tbsp peanut butter | 9 |
| 1 cup rice | 9 |
| 1 cup spaghetti | 5 |
| 1 cup cooked vegetables | 4 |
| 1 potato, baked with skin | 5 |
| 1 slice bread | 3 |
| 1 banana | 2 |

If a 150-pound woman ate one cup of yogurt in the morning, three ounces of tuna in a salad at lunch, and four ounces of chicken at dinner, she would consume 57 grams of protein, exceeding the 54 grams recommended for her. However, she consumed more than that because she also ate some bread, vegetables, and used some milk to lighten her coffee, all of which combined for an additional 20 grams of protein. Typical lacto-ovo American vegetarians consume about 100 grams of protein a day. These numbers indicate that if you want to try something a little different, which may help you reduce the fat content of your diet or control your weight effectively, consider experimenting with a lacto-ovo vegetarian diet. It is safe, interesting, and may be just the change of pace you need.

## Very Low-Calorie Diets (VLCDs)

Most overweight people have tried to fast at least once. This makes sense. Since weight control involves eating more than the body can use, why not eat nothing at all? Unfortunately, soon after beginning a total fast, the brain becomes very unhappy. This is an oversimplification but tells something of the story. The blood glucose levels decline, and the brain essentially commands the body to supply it with nutrients anyway. This demand results in the breakdown of lean body tissues, such as organs and muscles. The heart is essentially a muscle. What can and sometimes does happen during starvation is that the heart and other vital organs begin to "decompose." The body begins consuming itself as a desperate means to survive for another day. For a day or two, this may have little noticeable effect. However, if fasting persists for several weeks, the body becomes unable to function. Even for a single day, fasting leads to greatly decreased physical activity, light-headedness, dizziness, and other unpleasant symptoms. Fasting also does not work. People who fast for a day or two become ravenous and eat voraciously once the fast ends.

A much more modern and more useful version of fasting has developed during the past 20 years. One name for this approach is "protein-sparing modified fasting." The name for the modern version of fasting indicates that the body's protein supply (its organs and muscles) is not used as fuel during this type of fasting. Very low-calorie diets (VLCDs), another name for protein-sparing modified fasting, provide a maximum of 800 calories per day. The VLCDs that were popular 20 years ago included liquids composed of such poor sources of protein as cow- and horsehide. People drank these potions (for example, the Cambridge Diet) and received relatively low amounts of incomplete protein (approximately 30 grams per day or about half their normal requirements). At least 50 people in the United States died from their attempts at weight control using this inadequate VLCD. Today's versions include liquid fasts that provide about 70 grams of protein derived from high-quality sources of protein (usually egg whites and milk solids). Examples of these modern liquid VLCDs include Optifast, Medifast, and HMR (Health Management Resources).

Optifast and the other modern VLCD fasting programs are provided in clinics that include careful medical monitoring. The following protocol describes the lab work schedule for people who use Optifast in the program that I direct.

### Lab Work Schedule for Optifast

| Week | Tests |
| --- | --- |
| 0 | Chem-screen*, urinalysis, Electrocardiogram (EKG), full medical evaluation |
| 1 | Potassium (K+), uric acid, medical follow-up visit |
| 4 | EKG, K+, medical follow-up visit |
| 8 | K+ |
| 12 | EKG, Chem-screen*, medical follow-up visit |

*The tests marked with an asterisk require fasting for 12 hours before taking the test.

You can see that the use of liquid VLCDs requires a substantial commitment. The lab work takes time, costs money (often covered, in part, by insurance companies), and requires some unpleasant procedures (such as having blood drawn rather frequently). Liquid VLCDs also interfere with people's lives to a considerable extent. Consider the following comments by some of my clients over the past several years:

- "I never fully realized how much of our lives are spent eating together."

- "I found I became very isolated from other people."

- "I found it awkward during business lunches and dinners. Sometimes I brought my packet, mixed it, and drank it during meetings. It generated a lot more discussion than I wanted it to."

- "People were nice about it, but it made me feel weird and left out."

- "I longed for something I could crunch. Just broccoli or carrots or something!"

- "I started looking over food advertisements and longing for almost anything."

- "You never realize the pleasures of a simple hot meal until you live on cold milkshakes for a few weeks."

The commitment and difficulties of managing life on a liquid eating plan are worth considering before trying one. These approaches are recommended only for people who need to lose 40 or 50 pounds or more. In addition, a number of medical problems prevent people from using a liquid VLCD, including recent heart attack (within three months), history of circulatory problems, diabetes with a history of severe ketosis, chronic use of steroids (greater than 20 milligrams per day), bleeding peptic ulcers, history of suicide attempts or severe depression, and active problems with blood clots (or other conditions where decreased blood volume would put the individual at risk).

## Weight Loss on VLCDs

Evaluations of the effects of using liquid VLCDs are somewhat mixed, but promising. Use of liquid VLCDs seems to increase the rate of weight loss substantially for many people. For example, average weight losses after 12 weeks of fasting approach 50 pounds in many studies. However, approximately 50 percent of the people who complete 12 weeks of these programs regain substantial amounts of weight within a year and even more within two years. On the other hand, the other 50 percent maintain weight losses of 20 pounds or more at the end of a year, and approximately one-third of participants maintain weight losses of 40 pounds or more. Some studies show even greater promise than this. In an evaluation of the results of a program I have directed for the past 10 years, my colleagues and I found that participants who used a liquid VLCD maintained average weight losses of 34 pounds for 2 1/2 years after beginning the treatment program. While many people (perhaps a majority) cannot sustain fasting for the full 12 weeks, many others can do this with the appropriate kind of support.

If you are 40 pounds overweight or more, consider joining a professional program that uses a liquid fast. It is critical to remember, however, that the ingredients for long-term success include continued involvement in some type of supportive program. If the professionally conducted program does not provide continued individual or group support sessions, consider joining Weight Watchers or seeking the help of a professional therapist to sustain your focus in the long run. Very few people who need to lose 40, 50, or 100 pounds can sustain the focus that they need without some assistance. You can always try doing this on your own and then get help if you do not succeed. The key is to observe carefully the effects of any eating plan on your health and weight status. If the effects are less than what you want, it is time to take some other step.

## Recipe Suggestions for Optifast and Related Products

Optifast flavors include vanilla, chocolate, strawberry, orange, and cherry.

The following are general instructions for mixing:

1. Use a blender and drink immediately after mixing.

2. Mix packets with water, ice, and/or a variety of soda pops containing NutraSweet, such as the *diet* versions of cola, ginger ale, root beer, and orange.

3. Add flavorings to mixture. Non-caloric sweeteners may also be used. Flavorings are used in 1/8 to 1 teaspoon amounts. You might try:

| | | |
|---|---|---|
| Almond | Anise | Banana |
| Black Walnut | Brandy | Cherry |
| Chocolate | Coconut | Lemon |
| Maple | Mint | Orange |
| Peppermint | Pineapple | Root Beer |
| Rum | Sherry | Strawberry |
| Vanilla | Wintergreen | |

4. Freeze mixes into slushes.

Patients on Optifast contributed the following recipes. They all make one serving.

**Flavored vanilla Optifast**—Blend in mixer thoroughly:

- 3/4 cup cold water

- 1 tsp. any flavoring: peppermint, almond, chocolate, banana, vanilla, lemon, anise

- 1 packet vanilla Optifast or related product

**Orange dreamsicle**—Blend in mixer thoroughly:

- 1 can Diet Orange Crush

- 1 cup chopped ice
- 1 packet vanilla Optifast or related product

**Chocolate banana** Optifast—Blend in mixer thoroughly:

- 1 can diet fudge soda
- 1 packet vanilla Optifast or related product
- 1/2 teaspoon banana flavoring

**Boston coffee**—Blend in mixer thoroughly:

- 1 cup hot coffee
- 1 packet vanilla Optifast or related product
- 1 packet Equal sweetener

**Mocha moment**—Blend in mixer thoroughly:

- 6 ounces boiling water
- 1 teaspoon instant coffee
- 1 packet Equal sweetener
- 1 packet chocolate Optifast or related product

# Key Principles

- Diets don't work as a permanent method of weight control. Structured eating plans or diets, however, can help break patterns of problematic eating.

- If you can self-monitor everything you eat, you can control your weight.

- Among the suggestions in the "Almost Never" plan are to almost never eat fried foods, desserts other than fruit, and cheese (other than no-fat or very low-fat cheese). Almost always eat low-fat/low-sugar foods, low-fat/low-sugar snacks such as popcorn, pretzels, fruit, low-calorie cocoa, grilled fish and fowl, vegetables, mustard, salsa, and other spices on many different foods.

- The Popcorn plan encourages consumption of seven servings from proteins, five from breads and starches, two from fruits, and as many free vegetables and some miscellaneous foods as desired. It provides about 1000 calories per day and a low-fat eating plan (less than 20 percent of calories coming from fat).

- Vegetarianism (particularly lacto-ovo) provides yet another approach to healthful low-fat eating. No special efforts are required to get adequate amounts of protein if your plan simply includes eggs and dairy products.

- Very low-calorie diets (VLCDs) can help people who need to lose 40 pounds or more. I recommend trying one of the supervised medical programs, which provide appropriate medical screening and monitoring and group support. The key to maintenance of weight losses achieved via VLCDs is the same as the key to success through any approach at weight control: persistence. This may well include continued involvement in a program to help sustain your focus of attention.

# Epilogue

## Weight Controllers' Top Ten Rules for Dieting in a Saner, Fairer World

10. Food consumed for medicinal purposes doesn't have any calories. This includes throat lozenges, cough drops, chicken noodle soup, and anything bought in a Jewish deli (especially pastrami on rye sandwiches).

9. Using sugar substitutes in coffee entitles you to a free dessert every once in a while. Every once in a while includes two Fridays on either side of your birthday and every Saturday night except for the second Saturday in February.

8. Snacks consumed after midnight don't count because "it could have been a dream, anyway."

7. Pieces of cookies, bagels, and cheese (not cubes or slices) have no calories. The process of breaking uses more calories than the pieces contain.

6. If you drink a diet soda with pretzels or popcorn, the pretzels and popcorn have no calories. First of all, pretzels and popcorn are good low-fat snacks, anyway. Second, the calories in these good snacks are canceled by the diet soda.

5. If you eat with someone else, the calories you consume don't count if you eat less than they do.

4. Foods that have the same color have the same number of calories, for example, tomato sauce and cherry pie, yogurt and cheesecake.

3. Tasting food while preparing it is not really eating. Licking peanut butter off the knife while making a sandwich for your son or daugh-

ter is necessary to ensure the adequacy of the peanut butter, and therefore, no calories are consumed during this important parental task.

2. If you eat something very quickly and/or if no one sees you eat it, it has no calories. Maybe it never happened?

1. Snacks eaten at movies or theaters (for example, Milk Duds, buttered popcorn, Tootsie Rolls, chocolate bon bons) have no calories because they are part of the entire entertainment package.

# 6

# Effective Exercising

## A Long Climb to Success

Steve Silva's tears told the story. The ordeal was over. Steve had just completed a heroic assault on the world record for the vertical mile. He had raced up and down the Eiffel Tower 7 1/2 times, covering a heart-thumping 9127 steps in 2 hours, 2 minutes, and 54 seconds.

Steve finished just 1 1/2 minutes shy of the world record. "I wasn't crying because I didn't make it," said a smiling Silva a few minutes later. "I was just so glad to finish!" By finishing, Steve Silva achieved a much longer climb than the Eiffel Tower. Eight years prior to that moment, Silva weighed 435 pounds. Silva, a 39-year-old high school teacher, had lost 100 pounds six different times, only to gain it all back and more each time. Silva had ankle problems that made jogging and some other forms of exercise impossible. So he decided to climb stairs. Silva lost 245 pounds (down to a trim and powerful 190 pounds) by climbing up and down 30,000 steps a week.

Silva said his weight still fluctuates, but now "I eat more, but more veggies. I've learned to have more undereating weeks than overeating weeks." He advises others, "Make some reasonable changes; don't expect miracles." This is good advice from a man who has had more experience than almost anyone with life's ups and downs.

## Exercise Facts and Fictions

How much do you know about exercising? Most weight controllers accept its importance, but many confusions about it remain for many people. Please take the following "Exercise Test," and use it to evaluate your current knowledge.

# Exercise Test

*Circle the best answer for each question.*

1. Exercise doesn't promote weight loss as much as most people think; it takes a lot of exercise to burn off a few calories.    *True    False*

2. Sit-ups can help you lose fat from the midsection of your body.    *True    False*

3. Swimming does not help people lose weight.    *True    False*

4. Overweight people do not have underactive metabolisms.    *True    False*

5. Increasing daily activities (such as climbing more stairs and walking farther from parking places) does not help people lose weight.    *True    False*

6. Running three miles burns the same number of calories as walking those three miles.    *True    False*

7. Women and men burn the same number of calories when they do the same activities.    *True    False*

8. Jogging five miles per day every day of the week is the ideal exercise regimen for most people.    *True    False*

9. Exercise can increase appetite.    *True    False*

10. Exercise cannot affect bones and posture.    *True    False*

11. If you exercise at the level of your maximum heart rate for more than five minutes, you may die.    *True    False*

12. It is impossible to maintain the same level of cardiovascular fitness in your sixties that you had when you were in your twenties.    *True    False*

13. Weight lifting is appropriate for people under 40, but it presents too many risks for those who are middle-aged or older.    *True    False*

14. Exercise can improve cholesterol levels.    *True    False*

15. Exercise can improve resting metabolic rate.    *True    False*

## The Exercise Test: Answers and Explanations

1. *False:*    Exercise does promote weight loss at least as much as most people think. First, you expend significant amounts of calories during the exercise itself. For example, a fast walk for about 40 minutes burns off 200 calories. Second, you expend calories after the walk stops. That is, to replenish the energy consumed during exercise, the body must work harder than it does when it is resting. This increases metabolism.

Metabolism is the energy expended by the body to maintain itself (for example, by breathing, by digestion, excretion, and so on). Metabolism (or metabolic rate) may remain higher than normal for up to 24 hours after exercising. This means that the energy expended by exercising may increase substantially throughout the rest of the day after the exercise is completed. This increase in energy expenditure may amount to doubling the initial amount of calories burned off during the exercise.

Third, energy expended during the exercise and by elevating metabolism accumulates day by day, week by week. For example, the 40-minute fast walk, if completed every day, may amount to as much as one pound lost per week. That's 50 pounds per year. Fourth, exercising helps reinforce commitment to weight control. When people exercise, they think, "Why am I out here sweating when I could be home sleeping?" Then they remind themselves, "I'm out here because I want to control my weight, to look good, to be healthy. I'm here because I'm taking charge of this thing."

2. *False:*    Sit-ups cannot help you lose fat from your stomach (midsection). "Spot reduction" simply doesn't work. Your body takes fat supplies from places that it is directed to by your hormones and genetics. However, sit-ups can improve muscle tone. This could allow you to improve your posture and the appearance of your midsection. You can do this without consciously holding in your stomach. In addition, the improvement in muscle tone from sit-ups and related "crunches" can decrease back problems. When you improve muscle tone in the front and sides of your body, you place less pressure on your back (particularly the lower back). Since 80 to 90 percent of adult Americans develop some back problems (and even a higher percentage of obese people develop these problems), the benefits of sit-ups and crunches are clear.

3. *False:*    Swimming can help people lose weight. A recent study received a lot of attention because it seemed to show that swimming did not help people lose weight. However, this study was

flawed; there are many other ways of explaining the results. The biological reality is that any energy expenditure helps people lose weight. Swimming places less strain on the back, knees, and other weak parts of the body. If you swim approximately 20 yards per minute, you will expend approximately 100 calories in about 25 minutes. If you sit down for 25 minutes, you'll expend approximately 25 calories—that is, about 20 percent of the calories burned when swimming at that slow pace. If you swim at 50 yards per minute, for example, you'll expend 100 calories in about 8 minutes. That's about ten times more calories burned than by sitting.

4. *False:* Some overweight people do have underactive metabolisms. Metabolic rates vary just as all biological functions do. Some people are very efficient and expend relatively few calories to keep themselves functioning. Other people are much more inefficient and expend far more calories to keep themselves breathing, digesting, and staying alive. Exercise can increase metabolic rates.

5. *False:* Increasing daily activities (such as climbing more stairs and walking farther from parking places) can help people lose weight. Any expenditure of energy can help promote weight loss. You may recall the energy balance equation discussed in Chapter 4. When you expend more energy than you take in, you lose weight. You expend energy every minute of your life. If you are sitting down or watching television, you expend about one calorie per minute. As soon as you stand up, you burn two calories per minute. When you start moving around a little bit, you burn three calories per minute. If you start running, energy expenditure may go up to ten calories or more per minute.

Recently one of my newer clients came to a session eager to report on her increase in exercise. She joined an aerobics class and began going to it three times per week. She also discussed her other activities. It turns out she also began gardening recently. She spent a few minutes calculating the number of calories expended during a recent weekend's gardening.

She gardened for approximately four hours on both Saturday and Sunday of that weekend. Based on her weight and the calories expended per minute in those activities, calculations showed that she burned approximately 2000 calories per day by gardening on both Saturday and Sunday. In contrast, her low-impact aerobics class probably resulted in an expenditure of only 300 calories per class. This means that one afternoon's gardening accounted for greater expenditure of energy than all three aerobics classes in that week! She was amazed. She had lost three pounds that week and attributed that sizable weight loss to the aerobics classes. Her gardening actually accounted for much more of the weight loss than did the aerobics classes. The lesson here is that whenever you have the opportunity to move, take it.

6. *True:*    Running three miles does burn approximately the same number of calories as walking those three miles. For example, when a 154-pound man runs at an 8-minute-mile pace, he will expend 100 calories in approximately 7 minutes. If that same man walks at a 17-minute-mile pace, he will expend the same 100 calories in approximately 14 minutes. This man could walk the first mile in about 17 minutes and then run the second mile in about 8 minutes (25 minutes total). If he did this, he would expend approximately 200 calories. He could also walk those two miles in 34 minutes and burn the same 200 calories.

       Running provides the advantages of expending the calories in a lot less time, and it may produce a longer-lasting increase in metabolic rate for several hours or so. Walking has the advantage of being less painful to do. Walking also produces fewer injuries to knees and backs, for example, than running. I have had quite a few clients who lost a lot of weight using running as their primary exercise. I have had even more clients lose weight using walking as their primary exercise. For example, one of my clients lost 250 pounds doing no other exercise than fast walking (approximately 40 minutes per day).

7. *False:*    Since most men weigh considerably more than most women, women and men usually do not burn the same number of calories when they do the same activities. If a man and a woman weighed the same amount, they would burn approximately the same number of calories doing the same activities. For example, a 154-pound person would take 10 minutes to expend 100 calories when running a 12-minute mile. A 128-pound person would take 12 minutes, running at that same pace, to burn 100 calories.

8. *False:*    Jogging five miles per day every day of the week is not the ideal exercise regimen for most people. Jogging is a wonderful form of exercise. It is efficient and it produces many benefits. However, jogging pounds the knees, jars the hips, crunches the spinal column, and creates a variety of back problems. The risk of knee, back, hip, and other injuries increases substantially if someone jogs more than five days per week. These orthopedic risks also increase substantially when people jog for more than 30 minutes per outing. Since almost everyone would take quite a bit more than 30 minutes to jog five miles, the combination

of jogging five miles plus jogging seven out of seven days creates a substantial risk for injury.

Overweight people in particular would be ill advised to attempt such a regimen. Excess weight creates excess pounding on the knees and increases the likelihood of foot, hip, and back problems. Walking seven days per week, on the other hand, would create few such problems.

9. *True:*   Exercise can increase appetite. Mild to moderate exercise can *decrease* appetite substantially. For example, most people find they desire food less if they exercise 10, 15, 20, and even 60 minutes. However, exercising for several hours often *increases* appetite substantially. You can prevent this increase in appetite by eating or drinking beverages with calories during extended periods of exercise. Liquids are easiest to digest during exercise, and carbohydrates are also relatively easy to digest. For example, fruit juices and fruit make good appetite suppressants during extended exercise.

10. *False:*   Exercise can affect bones and posture. After about age 35, bone mass (sometimes called bone density) gradually decreases. This bone loss can lead to osteoporosis, the creation of fragile bones that break and bend easily. Exercise preserves bone mass or density.

Consider what happens when adults stay in bed (for example, during illness or hospitalization). They typically lose as much bone mass in two weeks as they would normally lose in a year. Studies have shown that exercising regularly can actually build bone in older people. One such study showed an increase in bone mass in a group of women whose average age was 81.

11. *False:*   You can exercise at the level of your maximum heart rate for far more than five minutes without any concern about dying. You could actually survive at your maximum heart rate for many days. This principle holds unless you have a heart condition.

12. *False:*   It is very possible to maintain the same level of cardiovascular fitness in your sixties that you had when you were in your twenties. Remember your hunter-gatherer ancestry. Hunter-gatherers maintained high levels of activity throughout their lifetimes. People in industrialized countries maintain high levels of activity during childhood (at least most people do), but they become more and more sedentary as they get older. Inactivity begets weakness; weakness begets injuries and more weakness. Studies show that regular aerobic exercise can maintain cardiovascular fitness and can even reverse some of the

damage done by sedentary living. For example, in a recent study, 19 men and women in their sixties exercised aerobically for about one hour three times per week. After two months, their resting metabolic rates increased by about 10 percent (on average), virtually eliminating the decline in resting metabolic rate of their entire lifetimes.

Aerobic capacities, or fitness levels, can also improve radically with persistent exercise. Many reports testify to the remarkable conditioning of runners and other committed athletes who were measured in their youths and then again in old age. Very few declines in aerobic conditioning occurred for these athletes. As people grow older, reflexes slow down and some decreases in flexibility seem almost inevitable. But cardiovascular fitness can be maintained at very high levels. Sixty-year-olds can, indeed, have cardiovascular systems like 20-year-olds. The table on the following pages documents this point quite dramatically. (The table is reprinted, with permission, from the September 1992 issue of *Self* magazine.)

13. *False:* Weight lifting is very appropriate for people of all ages. With proper supervision, even 90-year-olds can benefit from weight lifting. For example, a study with ten 90-year-olds had them lift weights with their legs for 10 to 20 minutes, three times per week. After eight weeks, they could lift three times more weight than they could prior to beginning weight lifting. Two of the nonagenarians gave up their canes after just eight weeks of lifting.

14. *True:* Exercise can improve cholesterol levels. Some evidence suggests that regular exercising can increase the level of HDL, or "good cholesterol."

15. *True:* Exercise can improve resting metabolic rate. You may recall the term "adaptive thermogenesis" mentioned in Chapter 2. When people decrease their food intake, metabolic rates usually decline. Adaptive thermogenesis involves changes in your metabolic rate. Metabolic rate refers to the rate at which your body uses (metabolizes) energy when you are resting. Your body uses quite a bit of energy even when you rest in order to digest food, keep you breathing, and so on. Studies with both animals and humans clearly show this effect. Your body slows down your metabolic rate when the food supply becomes scarce. This would allow you to survive during food shortages (when the hunting and gathering is not going so well). If you exercise regularly, your body reacts as if everything is okay. If you are moving around a lot, your body "knows" you must not be starving.

# Only the Fit Stay Young: Changes in Women's Bodies at 20, 30, 40, 50, 60, and 70

## Twenties

### The Fit Woman

. . . she retains the strength, stamina and flexibility of her teen years. Her leanness allows the definition of her muscles to show through. Late in this decade her bone strength may reach its peak. If she continues regular weight-bearing exercises, consumes plenty of calcium-rich foods, and gets adequate caloric intake, her bones will stay healthy for years to come. A lot of time spent outdoors without adequate sun protection will cause her skin to begin to freckle and develop very fine lines.

### The Sedentary Woman

. . . she may look great, but physical changes are already beginning to take place that could have far-reaching effects. Her aerobic capacity begins to decline at the rate of 1 percent per year. After age 25, muscle mass can decrease by an average of 5 percent every decade. Metabolism begins to drop at a rate of 2 percent per year, which will translate into increasingly higher body-fat percentages. Any fat added now will be distributed evenly throughout her body. She will begin to experience tightness in her hips.

## Thirties

### The Fit Woman

. . . she looks and feels as fit as in her twenties. She's agile and coordinated, with a lean, defined physique, thanks to well-developed muscles and below-average body fat, and her aerobic capacity—the ability to transport oxygen throughout the body—is better than ever. She will, however, begin to experience an unavoidable decline in the number of fast-twitch muscles, which are responsible for quick reaction time and for high-intensity activities like sprinting. If bone strength has not yet peaked, it will by age 35.

### The Sedentary Woman

. . . she will begin to feel her age in terms of muscle strength, particularly in her arms and legs. This is because her muscle fibers are starting to atrophy, and her muscle mass will continue to decline at a rate of about 6.6 percent each decade from here on out. She feels stiffer, as elastin is lost from her muscles. She could have as much as 33 percent body fat, most of it concentrated in her hips and thighs. Along with that of her active peers, her sexual responsiveness reaches a peak—but she may not have the energy to enjoy it.

## Forties

### The Fit Woman

... she remains as energetic and flexible as ever, with excellent aerobic stamina. Because of an inevitable decline in metabolism, however, she may have a tendency to put on some fat—particularly in her hips and thighs. But her high ratio of muscle-to-fat keeps her calorie-burning capacity up, and this, along with continued aerobic exercise, will counteract this tendency, keeping her at about 22 percent body fat. Although she experiences some compression of the vertebrae in her back, strong muscles keep her stomach relatively flat, her back supple.

### The Sedentary Woman

... she is by now 15 percent weaker than she was in her thirties, and the decline will be even more dramatic past age 45. Her shoulders appear narrower as muscle mass decreases in her upper back. The disks between her vertebrae begin to compress, so that with time she will be 1 to 1 1/2 inches shorter, and her stomach will distend as the distance between her ribs and pelvis decreases. She has lost about 40 percent of the range of motion in her hips and may develop varicose veins.

## Fifties

### The Fit Woman

... she has maintained every aspect of fitness. Her age shows only in her percentage of body fat, which continues to increase slightly—it's probably up to about 24 percent now. Gravity may start to take its toll on her body, and she may feel some wear and tear in her joints due to years of activity. She may want to rethink her workouts, switching to lower-impact activities—swimming or walking, for example.

### The Sedentary Woman

... she has poor posture due to the continued drop in flexibility and muscle strength. She slouches forward, and has a protruding stomach and overarched lower back. All the repercussions of inadequate aerobic activity begin to kick in: Her blood pressure rises; she becomes more susceptible to diabetes and heart attacks. Now body fat begins to settle around her middle, her skin wrinkles and is tugged downward by gravity.

## Sixties

*The Fit Woman*

... she has strong, flexible muscles and plenty of stamina. Despite the effect menopause has on estrogen production, her bones are strong, thanks in part to the weight-bearing exercises and strength training she's done all her life (although hormone replacement may be necessary). Her target heart rate will be about 115 beats per minute (down 30 or 40 bpm from her twenties). But because aerobic exercise has kept her heart strong, she remains able to pump healthy amounts of blood. She has about 26 percent body fat.

*The Sedentary Woman*

... she is two or three inches shorter by now and may have developed osteoporosis, partly because she has not done the weight-bearing exercise that keeps bones strong. Her breasts begin to sag in earnest and her waist widens even more. Her heart is 10 to 15 percent weaker than it was when she was 20, and measurable changes in her immune system increase her risk of developing cancer and certain infections. Wrinkles are now creases, and skin is dry.

## Seventies

*The Fit Woman*

... she can work and play almost as hard as she did 30 years ago. Only a slight increase in body fat—amplified by the earth's pull—reveals her age, along with deeper creases in her face and a drier look to her skin due to a decline in oil production that occurs after menopause.

*The Sedentary Woman*

... she is in failing health as high blood pressure, brittle bones, and unhealthy blood cholesterol levels leave her vulnerable to a host of serious diseases. Her flexibility, strength, and stamina are about nil, and she may have developed the classic "dowager's hump." She has wrinkles in her cheeks, and her mouth turns down, so she appears as unhappy as she probably feels.

Again, studies with both animals and humans show that exercise can reverse this slowdown of the metabolic rate. This important effect means that your body will expend more energy when you are not exercising and will allow you to lose weight more easily.

## Benefits of Exercising

The exercise test makes it clear that exercising is critical for effective weight control. Steven Blair also made this point with his "Exercise Quiz," published in 1991 in *The Weight Control Digest.* You may improve your commitment to exercising if you list the many ways exercise can affect you. While you know exercise can improve your ability to control your weight, can you list 10, 20, or 30 reasons to exercise regularly? Perhaps the following list of 50 benefits of exercising will help you make a clearer and stronger commitment to exercising. When reviewing this list, consider how each benefit could affect you. Exercise can:

1. Increase weight loss
2. Improve maintenance of weight losses
3. Improve stress management
4. Improve the quality of sleep
5. Improve digestion
6. Enhance self-esteem
7. Improve resistance to illnesses
8. Help you feel energized
9. Promote better digestion and bowel functioning
10. Tone muscles
11. Provide more definition to muscles.
12. Reduce blood pressure
13. Reduce tension
14. Improve flexibility
15. Build strength
16. Promote greater endurance
17. Decrease the negative effects of aging
18. Decrease menstrual cramping
19. Increase metabolic rate
20. Enhance coordination
21. Improve posture

22. Decrease back problems and pain

23. Decrease resting heart rate

24. Strengthen bones and joints

25. Improve reaction time

26. Strengthen the heart

27. Prevent heart disease

28. Improve cholesterol levels

29. Prevent osteoporosis (weakness of the bones)

30. Decrease the risk of cancer (particularly from colon cancers)

31. Improve abilities to relax more quickly

32. Decrease depression

33. Increase emotional stability

34. Improve quality of thinking

35. Improve ability to stay warm in colder climates

36. Improve ability to tolerate warmer climates

37. Improve agility

38. Improve body image

39. Increase endorphins (internally produced opiates that improve feelings of well-being and mood)

40. Decrease constipation

41. Improve social life (for example, by meeting new people during exercising

42. Improve athletic performance

43. Increase life span

44. Increase feelings of control or mastery

45. Improve rosiness of complexion

46. Decrease appetite

47. Provide balance in life

48. Increase self-awareness

49. Provide time to think, gain perspective, and solve problems more effectively

50. Promote self-actualization

This is a rather convincing list, isn't it? Many of the benefits of exercise pertain directly to weight control. Changes in muscles, bones, fat, and attitude can all affect success at weight control. Exercise must become a major part of your life if you plan to persist effectively at weight control. In fact, some studies of successful weight controllers show that virtually no one succeeds at weight control who does not become a frequent exerciser. Some of these studies included people who lost 50 pounds or more and maintained it for more than five years. Only 20 percent of Americans over 25 years old exercise at least twice per week. Almost 100 percent of successful weight controllers exercise more frequently than that.

## Can Exercise Prevent Cancer?

Seventy years ago, two Minnesota physicians noticed that most of their patients who developed cancer led sedentary lives. They also noticed that farmers they knew rarely developed cancer. They speculated that hard work and physical activity might prevent cancer. They compared cancer rates among various occupations. As they expected, cancer rates decreased as physical activity increased.

More recent research has supported the idea that exercising regularly can prevent cancer. A study of 13,000 people conducted by the Institute for Aerobics Research in Dallas used the treadmill test to measure fitness levels and then track cancer rates over eight years. They found that men who were the least fit had more than 4 times the overall cancer rates than the most fit men. The least fit women had 16 times higher death rates due to cancer than the most fit women.

Exercising probably decreases cancers of the colon, breast, and prostate. Cancer of the colon is the second leading cause of death (next to lung cancer) in the United States. Fifty thousand Americans die each year from cancer of the colon. Twenty-one of 27 recent studies have found that as activity increases, rates of colon cancer decrease.

Exercise may prevent colon cancer by increasing the speed with which waste products get through the colon. Greater physical activity leads to greater mobility in the intestines, as well. Also, greater physical activity might affect some biochemical agents that promote increased speed of digestion. It follows that the less time waste products spend in the colon, the less time those waste products that contain cancer-causing substances (carcinogens) spend in the body.

An important study on breast cancer involved more than 5000 women who graduated from college between 1925 and 1981. The women who had been college athletes had about half the risk of breast cancer of nonathletes. Another study of 25,000 women in the state of Washington showed that those who had worked in physically active jobs had much lower incidences of breast cancer than those who had sedentary occupations. Exercising may prevent breast cancer because it lowers estrogen levels. Estrogen is a hormone that women have in relatively high quantities (much higher quantities than men).

Research on more than 17,000 Harvard alumni showed that among men over age 70, those who had remained most active had much lower incidences of prostate cancer than the least active men. However, the "most active" men expended more than 3000 calories per week in walking, climbing stairs, and playing sports compared to the least active men. It takes a lot of activity to expend 3000 calories. High levels of activity may decrease levels of the male hormone, testosterone. Lowering this hormone may decrease the risk of prostate cancer.

Frequent exercisers tend to have other habits associated with the decreased risk of cancer. For example, frequent exercisers smoke less and eat lower-fat diets than sedentary people. However, most of the studies on exercise and cancer did eliminate these factors when analyzing the effects of exercise. In other words, the studies found exercising reduces risks of getting cancer regardless of the effects of diet and smoking. It seems safe to conclude that exercising regularly can prevent cancer.

# How To Exercise for Effective Weight Control

## Recommendations

Is it advisable to exercise every day? Is it advisable to exercise for 20 minutes per day? 40? 60? 120? What kind of exercise produces optimal results for weight controllers: aerobic exercise, or weight lifting, or a combination of both? Do everyday activities like walking to a bus or shopping help people lose weight?

The American College of Sports Medicine (ACSM) has provided recommendations to answer these questions. ACSM consists of many of the world's premiere experts on exercise. Their most recent set of recommendations has become well accepted around the world as the basis for developing safe and effective exercising patterns. Let's review answers to commonly asked questions by considering five aspects of exercising and the ACSM recommendations that pertain to them:

- Frequency of exercise
- Intensity of exercise
- Resistance training (weight lifting)
- Mode of exercise
- Duration of exercise

### Frequency of Exercise

Since exercise is so critical to weight control, I strongly encourage each of my clients to exercise every single day if at all possible. This exercise can vary from walking to swimming to playing racquetball. When people become accustomed to exercising in some form every day, they seem to lose more weight and maintain weight losses more effectively.

This recommendation of seven days per week is somewhat unusual. ACSM recommends four to six days per week to maintain a good level of fitness. However, because of the many benefits for weight control, I recommend placing greater emphasis on exercise.

Setting a daily goal for exercising may improve your consistency. People who set a permanent, daily goal, may not use as many excuses to avoid exercising. If you adopted a five-day-per-week goal, you could say to yourself, "Today is the day I won't exercise. I'll exercise tomorrow." This kind of thinking allows for many reasons to skip days. Have you said to yourself, "I don't feel like it today," or "I don't have time today." If you commit thoroughly to a daily goal, it is more difficult to allow yourself to postpone what is so critical to your well-being.

Some of my clients have used an expression to capture this: "not exercising is not an option." They have found that exercising every day increases their commitment to weight control. Daily exercise also increases metabolic rate more effectively and improves concentration on persistence. Remember, you are pursuing something other than a general improvement in your health. You are combatting biological forces that are dead set against weight loss. This takes extraordinary effort and commitment.

### Intensity of Exercise

Intensity refers to how hard your body works during a certain length of time. In other words, more intensive exercise means that your body works harder for the 15 or 30 or 45 minutes during which you exercise. Intensity varies depending on your level of conditioning or fitness. For example, world-class marathoners can run three 8-minute miles in a row and fail to break a sweat. To the average person, this intensity of running would prove extremely challenging. For the non-runner's body, this intensity level would be very high. For the world class marathoner, this intensity is very low.

Intensity of exercise is measured in several ways. The simplest way to measure it involves heart rate. The average heart rate of a 45-year-old man at rest is about 72 beats per minute. During moderate exercise, this increases to 145 beats per minute. Maximum exercise may lead to a heart rate of 175 beats per minute. This man's heart generally pumps about 5 liters of blood per minute while he is resting. During heavy exercise, his heart pumps about four times that amount of blood (20 liters). His breathing rate goes from 12 breaths per minute to 43 breaths per minute. His systolic blood pressure goes from 120 to 200 (mmHg). These biological changes occur because the body consumes a lot of energy and a lot of oxygen when it works hard. The muscle cells consume energy in the form of stored sugar (glycogen, glucose), as well as fats. The consumption of this energy requires oxygen, which is also used quickly during intensive exercise.

Your heart has a maximum capability for pumping blood and helping your body function during intensive exercising. You can actually sustain your maximum heart rate for many hours and perhaps many days. However, this maximum rate is considered an upper limit from which you can judge the intensity of your exercising. Subtract your age from 220 to calculate your maximum heart rate. If you are 40 years old, your maximum heart rate is 180 beats per minute (220 − 40 = 180). When you exercise at high intensity levels (close to your maximum heart rate), you become exhausted very quickly. You also increase your risk of injury through sprains and strains. In contrast, when you exercise at 60 to 80 percent of your maximum heart rate (your "training heart rate"), you stress your system in a positive way. This level of overloading your cardiovascular system actually can increase your heart's ability to pump blood throughout your body. By exercising at this recommended training heart rate, your muscles become increasingly efficient at extracting oxygen from your blood. This increase in efficiency takes time. It usually takes several weeks of fairly frequent exercise to improve efficiency at extracting oxygen from the blood and strengthening your heart. Gradually, however, anyone who exercises at this training rate enough becomes an increasingly fit individual.

Sometimes the term "aerobic capacity" is used to describe this type of fitness. Aerobic simply means involving oxygen. When you become aerobically fit, you increase your heart's ability to pump oxygenated blood through your body, and you increase the efficiency of your muscles at extracting oxygen from your blood. The more fit you are, the more oxygen and fuel (glucose, fat) you can get into your muscles quickly. This allows your muscles to work hard for long periods of time without producing feelings of exhaustion.

The most important rule of thumb about intensity of exercise is: Keep the intensity low enough to allow yourself to exercise for at least 30 minutes per session. Many people make the mistake of exercising too intensely for their current fitness levels. As a result, they become tired and find exercise painful after only a few minutes. If you jog at a slow pace (12-minute miles), you expend about 10 calories per minute. If you walk at a moderate pace (20-minute miles), you expend about 5 calories per minute. Weight control depends on total amount of energy expended. If you can only jog for 5 minutes at the 12-minute mile pace, you expend only 50 calories during that exercise session. On the other hand, if you can walk for 30 minutes at the moderate 20-minute mile pace, you would expend 150 calories. You expend three times more energy by exercising at the lower intensity level. That's all that matters for weight control. *Ex-*

*pend energy in a way that you can tolerate it.* If you push the intensity too high, you will become frustrated and decrease your exercising. From a weight control perspective, intensity is much, much, much less important than consistency. If you exercise frequently enough and for reasonable amounts of time (durations), you can really benefit from exercising.

For a quick check of exercise intensity, review the target zones listed in the following table for people ranging in age from 20 to 90 years.

| Age | Target Zone (60-80%, beats/minute) | Maximum Heart Rate (100%) |
|---|---|---|
| 20 | 120-160 | 200 |
| 25 | 117-156 | 195 |
| 30 | 114-152 | 190 |
| 35 | 111-148 | 185 |
| 40 | 108-144 | 180 |
| 45 | 105-140 | 175 |
| 50 | 102-136 | 170 |
| 55 | 99-132 | 165 |
| 60 | 96-128 | 160 |
| 65 | 93-124 | 155 |
| 70 | 90-120 | 150 |
| 75 | 87-116 | 145 |
| 80 | 84-112 | 140 |
| 85 | 81-108 | 135 |

After six months or more of regular exercising, you can exercise up to 85 percent of your maximum heart rate. This level becomes safe after consistent exercising for many months. However, you do not have to exercise that hard to stay in excellent condition. To check your heart rate during exercise, take your pulse immediately after you stop exercising:

1. When you stop exercising, place the tips of your first two fingers lightly over one of the blood vessels on your neck (carotid arteries) to the left or right of your Adam's apple. Another convenient place to determine your heart rate (or pulse) is the inside of your wrist just below the base of your thumb.

2. Count your pulse for ten seconds and multiply by six.

3. If your pulse (heart rate) is below your target zone, consider exercising a little harder next time. If you are above your target zone, exercise a little easier the next time. If your pulse falls within your target zone, you're doing fine.

Remember, any exercise, even exercise below your target zone, helps promote effective weight control. This recommendation about target zones pertains to maintaining and improving cardiovascular fitness. You may also find it helpful to check your heart rate if your approach to exercise creates too much of a strain. You can check to see if you are in your target zone, and you will probably find that you feel quite uncomfortable when you exercise above your target zone. Decreasing the intensity of your exercising will allow you to exercise for 30 minutes or more.

### Duration of Exercise

The American College of Sports Medicine endorses exercise sessions lasting from 30 to 60 minutes. Many people have difficulty maintaining aerobic activities for 30 minutes or more. If you are one of these people, try starting with sessions that last 10 or 15 minutes. Two 15-minute sessions of exercise produce about the same benefits as one 30-minute session. In fact, from a weight control perspective, you enjoy better results from frequent exercise for shorter amounts of time compared to one long session.

Some confusing theories exist about the length of exercise sessions. One concerns "fat burning." It suggests that you won't "burn fat" unless you exercise for long periods of time. This assertion is wrong. When you begin exercising, you begin using calories immediately. The energy consumed by your body initially comes from glucose stored in the muscles. As you exercise for longer periods of time, your body begins dipping into its energy reserves (fat). However, your body must replenish the energy supply it uses. This means that when you consume energy in the form of stored glucose from the muscles, your body will use its stored energy supply to replenish the glucose taken from the muscles. It makes no difference whether you exercise for short bursts of 10 or 15 minutes or for longer periods of 30 to 60 minutes per session. You burn fat both ways.

One of my clients, Lisa, described how she began exercising for very short periods of time. She then gradually extended the duration of her exercise:

> I began exercising for 15 seconds at a time on my Schwinn
> Air-Dyne with the oversized seat. I just couldn't seem to
> stay on that thing for more than a few seconds at a time.
> Of course, I weighed 340 pounds when I started using it.

So I did 15 seconds three times a day. Then I was able to do it longer and longer every day. Now, 190 pounds later, I use my Air-Dyne for 30 to 40 minutes every morning. Sometimes I go to an aerobics class or do a fast walk instead. But I exercise every day, sometimes twice a day. It makes me feel reasonably good. Although, I must admit, I would quit it all in a second if I could find some other way of keeping healthy and keeping my weight down. Exercising like I do sure beats the alternative of being so big.

## Mode of Exercise

When I was growing up in Brooklyn, New York, jogging didn't really exist. If you saw a man running down the street, you knew someone else was chasing him. The term "running shoes" also did not exist. The idea of spending as much money for running shoes as some people spent on used cars still amazes me.

The world has changed a great deal in these last 40 years. Options for exercising are everywhere. Health clubs are no longer places for fanatics. They are commonplace in many communities—especially in urban centers. Almost everyone has not only heard of running shoes—everyone owns at least one pair. Joggers run everywhere. Exercise has become part of everyday life.

Which options produce the best outcomes for weight controllers? My clients ask about the benefits of stairclimbing machines versus treadmills. People wonder about exercise equipment they can buy for their homes versus equipment in health clubs. Personal trainers have become another controversial addition to the possibilities for exercising.

Research shows that three elements of exercising seem particularly helpful: convenience, appeal, and social aspects. First, *convenience* affects exercising. If you join a health club 20 miles from your home or 20 miles from work, would you really use it regularly enough? Most people would not. In fact, many health clubs advertise as aggressively as possible to get people to join. The clubs realize that most people will not use the facilities, and their greatest profit comes from people who join and then disappear. Certainly walking, jogging, and in-home exercising are very convenient for most people. When looking at health clubs, consider joining one that requires minimal transportation. If you can find one next door to your job or within walking distance from home, it may be the best buy for you.

Second, the *appeal* of an exercise routine affects your use of it. Do you like walking? Or do you prefer a more social and musical activity like aerobics classes? Perhaps if you can make a game of your exercising, you would pursue it more effectively. Some people like racquetball and tennis because they enjoy the competition and camaraderie of those sports. You can also make your exercising as enjoyable as possible. Research shows that people who walk or jog exercise more vigorously and consistently if they use a Walkman-type radio/cassette player. Some recent versions include push-button digital tuning that makes switching from station to station very easy. Setting up a treadmill at home is an art form in and of itself. It helps to use earphones connected to the television and to a CD player to provide a variety of distractions. Many people also exercise at home in front of a VCR while watching a rented movie.

More equipment means more money. These are dollars well spent for weight controllers. However, many people do not have enough dollars to spare to buy such high-tech distractions. Various versions of the Walkman-type radio/cassette players, on the other hand, cost very few dollars and last a long time.

Finally, *social* aspects of exercise can affect consistency. If you can walk with a friend or spouse, you may find walking far more enjoyable than solitary journeys. The "loneliness of the long distance runner" can make it difficult to remain enthusiastic about exercising on your own. In contrast some people like the time alone that exercise provides. I have heard many people say, "Let me run on that tomorrow morning." These runners use their jogging time to solve problems. Problem solving goes remarkably well when phones aren't ringing and people aren't knocking on the door. If you are one of those people who enjoys the company of others while exercising, social sports such as golf, bowling, and others can add an important dimension to exercising.

> Riding a bicycle outdoors affords healthy exercise, fresh air, and an ever-changing vista of nature. Riding an exercise bicycle affords healthy exercise, with perspiration, and a first-class view of the sofa or TV. No wonder some people need to be coaxed into riding a stationary bike.
>
> Still, Americans each year buy three million exercise bikes, making them the nation's most widely sold piece of home exercise equipment. According to a recent survey, 42% of *Consumer Reports'* readers own an exercise bike.

Obviously many people choose the option of exercising at home. *Consumer Reports* evaluates exercise equipment every few years. The November 1990 evaluation recommended several exercise bicycles for indoor use, ranging in price from $250 to $4000. The *Consumer Reports'* engineers also suggested that some "dual-action" exercycles (bikes that include movable handle bars to exercise the arms) provide relatively quiet and effective exercise. (These cost around $700.)

My clients tend to prefer treadmills over exercycles. While most of them own exercycles, few use them regularly. The people who own treadmills seem to use them more frequently. Unfortunately, *Consumer Reports'* engineers found that most lower-cost treadmills don't work very well. They tend to be noisy and break down regularly. You might have to pay as much as $1900 for a high-quality, relatively quiet, and reliable piece of equipment that should last for many years. Then, again, it does cost as much as a used car.

Another mode of home exercising involves the use of exercise video tapes. Many of the video tapes on the market contain inappropriate information and some offer potentially dangerous advice. Nicki Euloff and David Thomas are two physiologists (experts in exercise) who evaluated the ten top-selling video tapes several years ago. These experts found that four of the video tapes contain as little as five minutes of aerobic exercise. Two contain none at all. Several of the tapes do not include enough warm-up time. *All* the tapes that were studied include exercise that the experts strongly advised against. These exercises included "ballistic stretching without adequate warm-up." Ballistic stretching is sudden, jerky exercise designed to increase flexibility. "Static stretching" is vastly preferred because it increases flexibility by slowly stretching a muscle and holding it in that position for several seconds. "Ballistic stretching" can tear or strain muscles very easily. Many of the tapes also include overextension of certain regions of the spine and knee joints. More recent tapes have improved somewhat. For example, Cathy Smith has created several safer and more appropriate video tapes ("Cathy Smith: Starting Out," and "Cathy Smith's Winning Workout"). Generally, use exercise video tapes with caution.

### Resistance Training (Weight Lifting)

It is a little-known fact that by age 74 about one-third of all men and two-thirds of all women can't lift a gallon of milk (approximately ten pounds). The average adult loses about six or seven pounds of muscle every ten years until age 45, and then even more muscle per decade after that. Most people have one-third fewer muscle cells than they had at age 20. Also, the muscle cells of 70-year-olds are smaller than those of 20-year-olds. Aging, however, does not cause these declines in muscularity. Disuse and sedentary living cause this weakening of the muscles.

In 1990 the American College of Sports Medicine recognized and emphasized the importance of resistance training more than in any of their previous recommendations. Strength training of moderate intensity (50 to 60 percent of maximal lifting ability) provides important benefits. The ACSM recommends selecting exercises that incorporate many different body parts and different kinds of movements. They suggest performing lifting exercises continuously, using smooth, slow, and controlled motions. Maintaining good posture when lifting weights also helps avoid injury. Only the body part being exercised while lifting the weight should be in motion during a lift. Other body parts should be at rest and stationary when weight lifting. The May 1992 issue of *Consumer Reports'* "On Health Newsletter" answered several critical questions about strength training, which are discussed here.

*How many repetitions?* Eight to 12 repetitions improve both strength and endurance. Most exercise experts suggest that if you can lift the weight easily more than 12 times, it is time to add more weight. When you add more weight, go back to 8 to 12 repetitions per exercise.

*How many sets?* ACSM recommends using 8 to 10 different kinds of weight lifting exercises per set. If you only make time to do one set, you will still strengthen your muscles 70 to 80 percent as much as you would by doing multiple sets. A full set of 8 or 10 exercises, including warm-up time, can take as little as 15 minutes to do.

*How many workouts?* The ideal strengthening program includes three workouts a week. Squeezing in more than three workouts per week might slow the growth of your muscles. Muscles need a day off to recover from weight training. Interestingly, you can get about 75 percent of the maximum improvement available from weight lifting by working out only twice a week. If you don't have much time, even a single strengthening session per week helps far more than none at all. According to one study, a weekly workout can maintain current levels of strength for several months.

*What about strength training for the legs?* People who do aerobic exercises may not need strengthening exercises for the legs. Most aerobic exercises keep leg muscles in good shape. However, strengthening for the legs may improve your ability to run, play sports, or climb stairs. It can also help older people walk longer distances and may prevent knee and hip injuries.

*How much is enough?* To keep building strength, you must keep increasing the weights you lift. You can maintain a desired level of strength by simply maintaining 12 repetitions for a particular exercise. If you stop weight lifting, your strength will begin to fade within two weeks. After three to five months, you'll be back to where you started.

*What's the procedure for weight lifting?* Several guidelines can help prevent injuries and maximize the benefits of weight lifting. First, it helps to warm up for a few minutes by doing jumping jacks, jogging in place, and then doing stretching exercises. It helps to stretch your shoulders, lower back, calves, and front and back of the thighs. Stretch slowly and steadily to the point of tension, not pain, and hold the position for 3 to 30 seconds.

Second, breathe slowly and steadily during weight lifting. Holding your breath while tensing muscles can cause light-headedness and even fainting. Exhale as you either lift the weight or raise your body, and inhale as you return to the starting position. Third, perform the repetitions slowly. Each one should take about six seconds—two to lift and four to lower. Jerky movements can cause injury and soreness. Fourth, stop if your muscles hurt. The dictum "No pain, no gain" is both wrong and potentially dangerous. Your muscles should feel fatigued during the last repetitions, but you should not feel sharp or piercing pains in your muscles. If you do feel pain, stop the exercise immediately. Finally, cool down after you exercise by doing a few minutes of walking or light jogging, followed by stretching again.

Specific weight training exercises include curls, rolls, and modified push-ups. *Consumer Reports* publishes several books that include specific stretching and weight lifting exercises, including *Get in Shape, Stay in Shape* by Skip Latella, Winifred Conkling, and the editors of *Consumer Reports*, and *Physical Fitness for Practically Everybody* by Ivan Kusinitz, Morton Fine, and the editors of *Consumer Reports*. You can order these books and others directly from *Consumer Reports* by calling 800-272-0722.

It is also helpful to have a well-qualified personal trainer show you proper techniques and a range of weight lifting exercises to consider. Personal trainers should have master's degrees in physical education or exercise physiology and certification by the American College of Sports Medicine. Most health clubs have at least one or two people with these qualifications.

### Benefits of Weight Lifting

One of the great things about weight lifting is that the equipment is very inexpensive. Also, the exercises take only a few minutes to do several times per week. Another point worth considering is that approximately 50 percent of the muscles in your body are not exercised through usual aerobic activities such as walking and jogging. If you build muscles and improve muscle tone, you may increase your metabolic rate. This is an additional, very useful benefit to strength training. Higher metabolic rates can promote more effective and efficient weight loss.

## Maintaining Commitment

### *Setting Exercise Goals*

The first step in maintaining your commitment to exercise is to evaluate your current level of activity. The following "Exercise Survey" lists many common exercises or sports. The purpose of this survey is to find out what types of exercise you are *currently* doing. If you have engaged in any of these exercises during the past seven days, write down the total number of hours spent in each activity in the last week.

If you participate in any exercises that are not listed, specify these activities in the "Other" category, including the length of time you performed them.

Finally, you'll notice that some activities are listed under more than one category. Because several exercises (walking, bicycling, swimming) may be done at varying levels of intensity, consider this when entering the time spent, and do so in the appropriate list. Please complete the survey now.

To score the exercise survey, add the total number of hours for light exercise and multiply by 240. Then add the total number of hours for moderate exercise and multiply that total by 420. Next, add the total number of hours for heavy exercise and multiply that number by 600. Finally, add all three numbers to give you a total. The total you obtain by completing the survey tells you something about your current level of exercising.

---

# Exercise Survey

## Light Exercise
(Approximately four calories expended per minute)

| Total Hours (last week) | Activity |
| --- | --- |
| _____ | Bicycling (5 mph) |
| _____ | Bowling |
| _____ | Calisthenics (light) |
| _____ | Canoeing |
| _____ | Dancing |
| _____ | Downhill skiing |
| _____ | Golf |
| _____ | Horseback riding |
| _____ | Horseshoes |
| _____ | Softball |
| _____ | Table tennis |
| _____ | Volleyball |
| _____ | Walking (3 mph) |
| _____ | Other_____ |

## Moderate Exercise
(Approximately seven calories expended per minute)

| Total Hours (last week) | Activity |
| --- | --- |
| _____ | Badminton |
| _____ | Calisthenics (moderate) |
| _____ | Cross country skiing (moderate) |

---

| Total Hours (last week) | Activity |
|---|---|
| _____ | Cycling (9.5 mph) |
| _____ | Dancing (fast) |
| _____ | Fencing |
| _____ | Ice skating (moderate) |
| _____ | Roller skating (moderate) |
| _____ | Stationary cycling (moderate) |
| _____ | Swimming (slow) |
| _____ | Tennis |
| _____ | Walking (4.5 to 5.0 mph) |
| _____ | Weight lifting |
| _____ | Other |

### Heavy Exercise

(Approximately ten calories expended per minute)

| Total Hours (last week) | Activity |
|---|---|
| _____ | Basketball |
| _____ | Calisthenics (fast) |
| _____ | Cycling (12 mph) |
| _____ | Handball |
| _____ | Ice skating (fast) |
| _____ | Jogging |
| _____ | Paddle ball |
| _____ | Racquetball |
| _____ | Roller skating (fast) |
| _____ | Rowboating |
| _____ | Skipping rope |
| _____ | Squash |
| _____ | Stationary cycling (fast) |
| _____ | Swimming (moderate) |
| _____ | Other |

No one particular number provides the "correct" level of exercising. When trying to lose weight, the more exercising you do, the easier it is to lose weight. You can use the number you obtained as a starting point. You can set exercise goals like "2000 calories per week," "3000 calories per week," or "10 percent increase per week for four weeks." You can redo the survey in one month, three months, or six months, and see the degree to which you made some constructive changes.

The exercise survey also provides a way to judge activities. Calories expended vary considerably depending on your size and the intensity with which the activity is performed. For example, under "Heavy Exercise," the survey suggests that "fast" stationary cycling and "moderate" swimming burn ten calories per minute. Far more specific tables of energy expenditure are available. The most readily available and detailed of these lists is provided by James Rippe in *The Exercise Exchange Program.* The tables in this book indicate that a 154-pound man burns 100 calories in 8 minutes by swimming at a rate of 50 yards per minute. That same man would take 17 minutes to burn 100 calories if he swam 25 yards per minute. Consumption of calories through exercise increases by about 10 percent for every 15 pounds over that 154-pound benchmark. Most people do not need this level of detail to understand the range of calories expended in various activities. The exercise survey gives you a ballpark figure from which you can assess your progress.

You may wish to use a daily exercise record, such as the one presented on the next page. You can see that this form encourages entries for each day of the week (minutes of exercise). If you use this form, you could first record the exercise. Then indicate whether it was light, medium, or heavy by referring to the list of activities on the exercise survey. Next, enter the number of minutes of that exercise that you performed. Multiply the number of minutes by the calories expended per minute (light = 4, moderate = 7, heavy = 10). Then enter that total in the column, "calories used up." You could do this every day to judge your level of exercising for each week.

An alternative used more frequently by my clients involves self-monitoring of food. Using whatever form or booklet you use to monitor your food, simply enter exercise sessions at the top or bottom of the page each day. You could note the type of exercise you performed and the amount of time spent at it each day. If you find days in which no entries are made, it tells you that you are not reaching the daily goal. You could use this information to begin problem solving. If you accept the goal of trying to exercise every day, then self-monitoring of your exercise in this fashion could help maintain your commitment effectively.

# Daily Exercise Record

**Week of**_____ **through**_____

| Day | Exercise | L(4)  M(7)  H(10) | Minutes | Calories Expended |
|---|---|---|---|---|

1 _____

_____

_____

2 _____

_____

_____

3 _____

_____

_____

4 _____

_____

_____

5 _____

_____

_____

6 _____

_____

_____

7 _____

_____

_____

**Total Calories Expended This Week**_____

**Everything Counts**

Everyday activities aside from exercising also consume calories. The following are some common activities and the calories expended per minute by a 150-pound person:

| Activity | Calories Burned per Minute |
|---|---|
| Car washing | 4 |
| Gardening | 5 |
| Grocery shopping | 4 |
| Mowing lawn (pushing power mower) | 5 |
| Painting house | 5 |
| Raking leaves | 4 |
| Shoveling snow | 8 |
| Sweeping | 4 |
| Vacuuming | 3.3 |

You can see that many daily activities expend significant numbers of calories. These numbers confirm the dictum: Move whenever and wherever possible. If you want to lose weight and maintain weight loss, find creative ways of staying active. One of my clients did this by buying a desk that she could only use while standing up. She knew that standing burned twice as many calories as sitting and used this knowledge to her advantage. Another client who worked in a school decided to avoid the elevator in the school. She took the long way down corridors to talk to colleagues and students. People who work in stores can avoid escalators and use stairs whenever the alternative presents itself. Parking farther rather than closer to your destination provides additional opportunities for walking. Such everyday methods of expending calories really add up. Studies of overweight children in camp showed that they expended fewer calories playing the same games and sports as children who were not overweight. This indicates that people with weight problems may tend to avoid everyday activities more than those who do not have weight problems. Some recent studies of people in major cities also support this. When given the opportunity to take the stairs or an escalator or elevator, overweight people take the stairs even less than people who are not overweight. Every time you take a more active, rather than sedentary, alternative pathway, you burn calories and elevate your metabolic rate. Everything counts.

Some people select weekly goals for exercise expenditure. You can use the daily exercise record or some version of it to monitor your progress toward specific goals. I have found that monitoring exercise expenditure proves somewhat arduous for most people. It also seems unnecessary to monitor that level of detail. I recommend keeping track of whether or not you exercise each day, along with your self-monitoring of food. This degree of monitoring helps reinforce the goal of daily exercise. You may also wish to make a commitment to seeking opportunities to stay active as much as possible in your everyday life. This includes avoiding labor-saving devices whenever possible.

## Excuses, Excuses

I met one of my childhood friends for dinner last year. I had not seen Tom for 20 years. Tom looked good and was happy with his family life and work as a pharmacist. We talked about various things, including exercise. Tom noticed that I had lost a considerable amount of weight and seemed to be in excellent physical condition compared to the last time he saw me. He asked the usual questions about "my secret." I discussed the importance of exercise in my life. As a health professional, he was fully aware of the value of exercising. However, he told me, "I really wish I had time for exercise." I talked about the idea of making time for exercise rather than thinking of it as an option. He argued that he "just didn't have time for it." Upon further inquiries about this time constraint, Tom indicated that he believed exercise would interfere with his ability to earn a decent living. He wanted to work more and more hours every year to keep increasing his income. It turned out that he and his wife make a more than satisfactory income and have no major financial pressures. In fact, his wife is a successful physician and they earn more money than 99 percent of the households in the United States. I asked, "Wouldn't you and your family be better off if you were healthier and happier, than if you made an extra few thousand dollars per year by working additional hours that you could use for exercising?" Tom argued that he and his wife do not like to take out loans when they buy something like a car. I replied incredulously, "You mean that you feel a 'need' to pay for your cars in cash and that's the reason for avoiding exercise?" "I guess so," responded Tom weakly.

Exercise takes time and requires some sacrifice. Tom decided that the "sacrifice" of taking out a loan to buy a new car every ten years (which he and his family could easily afford) outweighed the benefits of exercising. This is a remarkable piece of rationalization. Most people do not have the luxury of paying cash for $20,000 cars no matter what they do. Instead, other ways of explaining lack of participation in exercise crop up all the time.

What are some of the ways you talk yourself out of exercising? The following is a list of thoughts that people sometimes use when they consider whether or not to exercise. Please read each thought carefully. Then, next to each thought, indicate how frequently you had that thought *during the past week*, using the following scale:

# Reasons To Avoid Exercising

*Frequency*                 *Reason*

_____    I'm too tired.

_____    I need more sleep.

_____    I have more important things to do.

_____    I'm too busy.

_____    I'd rather relax.

_____    I don't feel good enough.

_____    I'm just not motivated to do it.

_____    I'll do it tomorrow.

_____    I'll do it later.

_____    It's no big deal if I miss one day.

_____    **Total**

1 = Not at all

2 = Sometimes

3 = Moderately often

4 = Often

5 = All the time

If your total is 30 or more, you use excuses to avoid exercising quite frequently. Research conducted by Deborah Kendzierski and Wendy Johnson in 1993 showed that people who scored 30 or more on a similar questionnaire tended to exercise less frequently than those who reported using these excuses less often.

Take a look at each of these excuses and the disputing response that applies to it in the next table. You may think of other disputing responses that could help you. When you find yourself using an exercise excuse, consider disputing that excuse in some way. Feel free to use any of the suggestions in the table for disputing responses, or make up your own. By improving your awareness of the way you talk yourself out of exercising, you can improve your chances of talking yourself back into it.

| Exercise Excuses | Disputing Responses |
|---|---|
| 1. I'm too tired. | Exercising will energize me. I am unwilling to give in to a temporary feeling of tiredness. |
| 2. I need more sleep. | It would be nice to get more sleep. Exercising will help me sleep better. I can go to sleep earlier or sleep longer tomorrow. Being a little sleepy is not a major problem. |
| 3. I have more important to do. | Making time for myself is as important as anything else. I can work more efficiently if I exercise and stay healthy. I can even think about my work while exercising to jump-start it when I get back. |
| 4. I'm too busy. | What's more important to me? I can keep exercise as a high priority in my life. It does take time. It takes time to invest in myself, my health, my well-being. |
| 5. I'd rather relax. | Just because I'd rather relax doesn't mean that's the best thing for me to do now. I want to fulfill my commitment to improving my health and maintaining weight control. |
| 6. I don't feel good enough. | Unless I have a fever or I am deathly ill, I know it's safe for me to exercise. Perhaps I can exercise at a lower intensity than usual. I could walk instead of run, or I can jog slowly instead of at my usual pace. I can do at least 15 or 20 minutes of something. Even a reduced exercise session is better than none at all. It keeps me focused and increases my metabolic rate. |
| 7. I'm just not motivated to do it. | I don't have to wait for some magical level of "motivation." As they say in the Nike commercials, "Just do it!" If I think about why I want to exercise, that will increase my motivation or commitment. I know I'm committed to controlling my weight. Therefore, I'm committed to exercise. That commitment is motivation enough. |

| 8. I'll do it tomorrow. | I made time in my day to do it today. If I convince myself to do it later, I might not do it at all. If I get it out of the way, I'll feel better. I don't want to live like a procrastinator: "Why do it now, if you can put it off tomorrow?" |
|---|---|
| 9. I'll do it later. | If I can do it later, I can do it now. Why take the chance of missing an opportunity to exercise—an opportunity to meet my goals and satisfy my commitment. |
| 10. It's not a big deal if I miss one day. | Every day and every thing counts. If I don't make today count, what makes me think I'll make tomorrow count? My commitment is a commitment to every day. Every day counts. |

## Preventing and Managing Injuries

Was there any point in your life when you were a regular exerciser? What caused you to decrease your exercising? Injuries often interfere with exercise habits. When people injure their ankle or back, it can take a long time, if not forever, for them to get back to regular exercising. Even minor and common illnesses, including colds, can change the momentum of consistent exercising. Exercising takes time, costs money, and interferes with your life to a significant degree. When you are sick or injured, living without exercising becomes normal. This increases the challenge of working exercise back into a complicated life. This makes sense. There is nothing crazy or neurotic about not exercising. It takes devotion, commitment, and focusing to make exercising a part of your life.

You have choices about managing illnesses and injuries. First, you can either expect some injuries and illnesses to interfere with your exercising, or you can just hope "It won't happen to me." The latter hope almost never works well. You can plan more effectively when your expectations fit reality better. What will you do *if* you get sick? How would you manage a back or knee injury? It helps to plan for these common problems.

Second, you can take an aggressive approach to managing illnesses and injuries or a more conservative approach. The aggressive approach usually includes exercising sooner than you think you can. Doctors I've consulted often recommend resting when fevers go to 100 degrees or more. When fevers get below 100 degrees and you feel capable of some easy exercise, like walking, you can go for it. "Exercise a day or two before you think you can," I have heard from some very effective physicians. Consider your reaction to a doctor suggesting the more conservative (and typical), "rest until you're feeling much better." Do you simply follow that advice? You could. You could also challenge it gently by asking if you could go for a several-miles walk or some other workout sooner, rather than later.

Consider asking your doctor specifically about the medical risks of exercising at various levels of intensity and various durations. "Can I walk three miles? Five miles? Jog slowly three miles? Use a step machine for 20 minutes? Play doubles tennis?" "Yes" or "no" answers are not good enough. Try to find out advantages and risks of various alternatives. Then decide what to do. It's your body; your commitment to weight control. If you manage it as actively as you can, you'll probably feel better about it.

You can consult your doctor about illness and exercise, but who do you consult for some of the more common exercise-related maladies? Problems with knees, backs, hips, and feet plague middle-aged exercisers as well as many highly trained 20-year-old athletes. All athletic teams at the college level and beyond use athletic trainers to help mend these maladies quickly and avoid unnecessary damage. At Olympic events (Olympic Festivals, the Olympics), dozens of athletic trainers help the athletes stay competitive despite various strains and sprains. You can get similar assistance at physical therapy centers. Almost all hospitals have such centers. Sometimes these centers are located in hospital rehabilitation or orthopedic clinics.

Some large-scale studies also support the effectiveness of chiropractors, specifically for back problems. Sometimes foot problems lead to knee problems and/or hip and back problems. Podiatrists can help when feet become uncooperative.

Consider investigating physical therapy, chiropractic, and podiatric alternatives. Each approach has advantages and disadvantages, depending on the nature of the problem. The key to feeling better is—you guessed it—persistence. Try to pursue various alternatives until some approach makes sense and really helps. It is frustrating. The healing arts remain more art than science, unfortunately. Support from others sometimes helps, but even without support, remember the critical role exercise plays in effective weight control. You can find alternatives when injuries occur (walking or swimming instead of jogging or playing tennis, for example). You can refuse to stop moving whenever possible. You can manage your weight with an imperfect body. You cannot manage your weight by becoming sedentary.

### Safety Tips

Perhaps the best way of managing injuries is to avoid them. The American Heart Association suggests the following helpful hints:

- Stretch, warm up, and cool down.

- Build up your level of activity gradually.

- Listen to your body for early warning signs.

- Be aware of possible signs of heart problems.

- Take appropriate precautions for special weather conditions.

**Stretch, warm up, and cool down.** Warming up for several minutes gives your body a chance to get ready for more vigorous exercise. Start at a slow to medium pace and gradually increase it for several minutes. Warm-ups can include jogging in place or just moving around slowly beginning to orient your body to exercise.

Stretching exercises are a necessary part of the warm-up. Do stretching exercises slowly and in a steady rhythmical way. Many different stretches are possible. Here are four that are widely used:

- **Wall-push.** Stand one to two feet away from a wall. Lean forward, pushing against the wall, keeping heels flat. Count to ten, then rest. Repeat one or two times.

- **Palm touch.** Stand with your knees slightly bent. Bend from the waist and try to touch your palms either to your ankles or to the floor. Do not bounce. Count to ten, then rest. Repeat this one or two times. If you have lower back problems, do this exercise with your legs crossed.

- **Toe touch.** Place your right leg on a stair, chair, or other object. Keeping your other leg straight, lean forward slowly to touch your right toe with your right hand ten times. Then do this with your left hand ten times. Again, do not bounce. Switch legs and repeat with each hand. Repeat the entire exercise one or two times.

- **Shoulder blade scratch.** Reach back with one arm as if to scratch your shoulder blade. Use the other hand to extend the stretch. Alternate arms. Repeat one to two times.

Cool down for several minutes after exercising. The cool-down should progress slowly and gradually. For example, swim more slowly or change to a more leisurely stroke. You can also cool down by walking for several minutes after a jog. Cooling down allows your body to relax gradually. It also helps remove build-ups of the by-products of exercising that accumulate in the muscles. Abrupt stopping can cause dizziness and cramping or muscle soreness later in the day. Consider repeating your stretching and warm-up exercises to loosen up your muscles after an exercise session.

**Build up your level of activity gradually.** Starting out slowly helps avoid overexertion. This decreases the likelihood of injury. Remember, even if you walk at a slow pace, you accomplish much more than staying sedentary.

**Listen to your body for early warning signs.** You can feel pains in joints, feet, ankles, and legs quite easily when you're just getting used to exercising. Minor muscle and joint injuries can be treated readily by aspirin and rest. When you feel pain, discontinue what you are doing. If you feel a pain in your ankle when running, for example, try slowing down for a while and see if the pain goes away. If it persists, stop running. Some discomforts are perfectly normal during exercising. It may take a while for you to recognize the difference between normal discomforts and potentially problematic pains.

**Be aware of possible signs of heart problems.** Pain or pressure in the left or midchest area, left neck, shoulder, or arm during or just after exercising can be a sign of a heart problem. These sorts of pains can also occur due to the normal strains of exercising. For example, a "stitch" is a common, relatively sharp pain that occurs below the bottom of your ribs. It is a cramping of some muscles due to a temporary lack of oxygen to those muscles. Stitches stop when you slow down. Heart problems do not cause stitches. On the other hand, sudden dizziness, cold sweats, or fainting are signs of much greater concern. If any of these things happens during or immediately after exercising, get some medical attention right away.

**Take appropriate precautions for special weather conditions.** When it is hot and humid outside, consider exercising less than normal for a week or so until you adapt to the heat. It also helps to exercise during cooler parts of the day, such as early morning or early evening after the sun has gone down. If you recall the discussion on fluids in Chapter 4, you might remember that fluid intake becomes especially important under conditions in which you might become dehydrated (for example, when traveling or during particularly hot days). You do not need extra salt; you get enough salt in your diet. Also, if you maintain a good level of physical fitness, your body learns to conserve salt, and your sweat consists mostly of water.

On very hot and sunny days, the possibility of heat stroke is a concern. Signs of heat stroke include feeling dizzy, weak, light-headed, and excessively tired. Also watch for a sudden decrease in sweating, and a rapid increase in body temperature. If you feel sensations very much like these, get yourself to a cooler place as soon as possible, drink some fluids, rest, and seek medical attention.

Dress appropriately for hot weather. It helps to wear very light, loose-fitting clothing. Rubberized or plastic suits, sweatshirts and sweatpants do nothing but increase your risk of heat stroke. Such clothing does not help you lose weight any faster. It does make you sweat more, but the weight you lose in fluids by sweating is quickly replaced as soon as you begin drinking fluids again.

On cold days, wear one less layer of clothing than you would if you were outside but not exercising. Some people find that they can wear a couple of layers less than they normally would. Several layers of clothing work better than a single layer of heavier clothes. You can wear old mittens, gloves, or cotton socks to protect your hands. Some of my clients wear inexpensive cotton garden gloves while walking or running. Since up to 40 percent of your body's heat is lost through your neck and head, wearing a hat is especially advisable in cold weather. Hats made of "turtle fur" are particularly comfortable and do not itch as much as wool caps.

Remember that rainy, icy, or snowy days make for special hazards for exercisers. Persistent weight controllers develop a variety of alternative means of exercising that allow for these weather conditions. They may use indoor tracks or machines at health clubs, play racquetball, take tennis lessons, or use their own treadmills or exercycles. This is particularly necessary for those of us who live in climates like Chicago's.

**Other miscellaneous tips.** Here are a few additional hints for safe exercising:

- Avoid strenuous exercise for at least two hours after a meal. It also aids digestion to wait about 20 minutes before eating following an exercise session.

- Proper equipment can prevent a variety of injuries. This includes good running shoes for walkers or runners and goggles to protect eyes for racquetball, handball, or squash players.

- Hard and uneven surfaces such as cement or rough fields cause more injuries than smoother surfaces. Soft, even surfaces such as level grass fields, dirt paths, or tracks are better for your feet and joints.

- When you walk, run, or jog, try to land on your heels rather than on the balls of your feet. This minimizes the strain on your feet, knees, and lower legs. Try to keep your feet as close to the ground as possible without tripping. This method helps you land on your heels rather than on your toes.

- Walkers and joggers get hit by bicycles and cars more often than you might think. It helps to wear brightly colored clothes and reflecting bands on clothes and shoes. Drivers will notice you more if you face them. That also allows you to protect yourself more directly. The basic message is: exercise defensively. Bicyclists can prevent injuries by wearing a helmet, using a light, and putting reflectors on their wheels for night riding. It also helps to ride in the direction of traffic and to avoid busy streets.

One definition of middle age is: 15 years older than you are now. Forty years old represents another threshold for middle age that researchers use. Many people concerned about weight have crossed the magic 40-year-old threshold. Middle-aged weight controllers commonly experience minor injuries. Ankles get sprained, backs get painful, hips start hurting, and knees swell up. Every athlete experiences these problems as well. Remember that weight controllers are very much like athletes in training. You are attempting to push your body to a place it doesn't want to go. Your brain can take over and nudge your body forward, despite the inevitable aches and pains along the way.

## Exercise in Perspective

Sometimes persistence comes from taking stock. When you look back over the last five years, do you recognize any patterns in your exercising or lack of exercising? Were there times when you were very active? Did you become particularly sedentary after an injury? Have you generally had difficulty maintaining an effective exercise regimen? I've asked many of my clients to take stock of their exercising patterns this way. They report that this perspective sometimes helps them realize that patterns do exist. They may see patterns of inactivity followed by reassuring patterns of renewed efforts. Change never takes place in a straight line. Almost no one begins exercising, stays with one type of exercise forever, and never deviates. Consider the following exercise histories from two of my most persistent clients, Amy and Stuart. Do these histories match yours in some ways? As you read these, note the patterns of staying with it, refusing to give up, and willingness to try new or different things.

### Amy

1989, March - June:

– started walking program alone

– began walking in my neighborhood, one mile at first

– gradually built up to three to four miles per day

July - December:

– started walking with friends

– found that walking with friends made it much more enjoyable

– was able to increase frequency from two to three times per week to four to five times per week

1990, January - February:

– joined health club

- started playing racquetball
- didn't like it much

March - April:

- kept trying to play racquetball
- never really liked it
- couldn't quite get the hang of it
- tried swimming indoors
- it was okay, but I don't particularly like getting wet. I don't like the chlorine either.
- tried using the treadmill and liked that well enough

May - June:

- convinced my friend Leslie to join the health club
- we used the treadmill and walked on the track
- it was okay
- maintained good frequency, at least three times per week, sometimes five or six

July - August:

- injured knee (twisted it while stepping off the treadmill)
- got it evaluated and determined not to do anything dramatic
- found it difficult to regain momentum
- started gaining some weight
- felt depressed

September - December:

- began walking again by myself and with friends
- started using the health club when weather didn't permit out-side activity
- kept exercise frequency and intensity at good levels
- weight loss improved and I felt better about it
- still didn't like the exercising too much. But it worked.

1991, January - March:

- got into skiing for the first time. It was fun!
- I enjoy reading ski magazines and playing with the equipment.
- did a little too much drinking, but enjoyed the activity

– finally a way to make winter more tolerable

– nice to tie activity into enjoyment

April - December:

– got into walking again by myself and with friends

– took some aerobics classes at the health club

– they were okay

– exercise interrupted when I got the flu (but only for two weeks)

1992, January - April:

– enjoyed skiing again

– went on three trips this year!

– they were fun and I'm getting better at it

– I seem to have more endurance this year

– the skiing helped motivate increased intensity of workouts during the winter at the health club

May - June:

– used a personal trainer to begin weight lifting

– seems to help improve muscle tone

– it doesn't take much time

– I'd rather not do it, but it seems worth doing

July - December:

– back into walking with friends and by myself

– tried some swimming outdoors when weather permitted

– it was okay

– I still don't like getting wet

– went on two "charity walks"

– I was amazed I could do a six-mile walk pretty comfortably.

1993, January - December:

– pretty similar to 1992

– used a trainer sometimes

– continued some weight lifting and added some equipment for using at home

– trying to improve my stretching exercises

– developed a back problem

– got some help through a physical therapy clinic

– changed my stretching and warm-up routines to help back

– got moving as soon as possible this time

– it's going okay

## Stuart

1990, January - April:

– joined health club

– started using the treadmill; started at a very slow pace (2.5 mph, no elevation); gradually increased from 10 minutes to 40 minutes

– made a routine out of the club and the treadmill

– got up early (6:00 A.M.), to the club by 6:30, finished workout and shower by 7:45

– as weather improved, began walking outside with a Walkman

May - August:

– increased walks on weekend to one-plus hours

– took some two-hour marathon walks

– got into some bike riding, as well

– joined a coed softball team

– had fun with the softball, not sure about exercise value. More exercise than being a couch potato.

September - October:

– back went out!

– very painful, could barely move or sit. Got help from a chiropractor.

– added stretching exercises and warm-ups to working out

– back started feeling much better after several weeks

November - December:

– back to 30 to 40 minutes on treadmill each day

– increased speed to 4.5 mph

– added three degrees elevation

– found using Walkman on treadmill makes time go faster

1991, January - April:

– added some weight lifting to my routine

– lift weights two to three times per week for about 15 minutes

– starting to use the Stairmaster, to break the routine of the treadmill

May - August:

– again, walking program outside

– stopped using the health club and discontinued membership

– bought dumbbells to continue weight lifting at home

– found out that even rain doesn't have to stop you from exercising

September - December:

– invested in Gore-tex running suit

– cold weather doesn't bother me much now

– started increasing speed of my walks to slow jogs

– got new running shoes to decrease soreness in feet

1992, January - March:

– joined another health club very close to home

– it's good to have an alternative on icy days

– used the running track at the club, in addition to Stairmaster and sometimes treadmill

– started playing a little racquetball

April - August:

– back outside for the warmer weather

– slow jog has increased to nine-minute miles

– jog three to four miles five days a week now

– continue weight lifting and stretching routines

– played a little golf

September - December:

– continued stretching, weight lifting, and jogging

– went back to the health club to work with a personal trainer for a few sessions

– developed new weight lifting routine

– continue to see chiropractor every month or so; seems to be helping

1993, January - December:

– similar routine to 1992

– playing racquetball one to two times per week, though

– enjoy the company and the workouts

– the game motivates weight lifting and other exercise

– bought Stairmaster and set it up in basement

– set up Stairmaster with VCR and earphones

– good alternative to outdoor workouts when raining or icy

# Key Principles

- Exercise is critical to effective weight control. Many confusions exist about how exercise contributes to weight control. For example, many people mistakenly think that they can lose fat from their midsection by doing sit-ups. People also underestimate the very real benefits of increasing daily activities (such as climbing more stairs and walking). Another important fact pertains to the rate at which calories are burned (expended) through exercise. Running three miles and walking three miles burn similar numbers of calories.

- You may increase your commitment to exercising by carefully reviewing and thinking about the many benefits that exercise provides. Among those benefits are improved stress management, improved quality of sleep, improved digestion, decreased back problems, improved cardiovascular fitness, and decreased risk of cancer.

- The American College of Sports Medicine (ACSM) has made some important recommendations pertaining to the frequency, intensity, duration, and mode of exercising. My recommendations are based on ACSM's guidelines: (1) *frequency:* exercise daily; (2) *intensity:* keep intensity low enough so that you can tolerate exercising for at least 30 minutes; it improves cardiovascular fitness to exercise at 60 to 80 percent of your maximum heart rate; (3) *duration:* 30 to 60 minutes per exercise session; two 15-minute sessions provide similar benefits to one 30-minute session; all energy expenditure helps burn fat; (4) *mode:* select modes of exercising that are convenient, that have appeal to you (that you like), and consider options for exercising that involve other people; (5) *resistance training (weight lifting):* consult a certified athletic trainer or review some of the available written materials to select 8 to 10 weight lifting exercises to use; complete 8 to 12 repetitions per exercise, and complete three sets three times per week to obtain maximum benefits.

- Exercise goals can include 1000 calories expended per week or any other level you select. You may find it useful to monitor calories expended in exercising. "Light" exercise expends approximately seven calories per minute (for example, cross-country skiing, bicycling at 9.5 miles per hour, fast dancing, and stationary cycling at a moderate pace). "Heavy" exercise expends approximately ten calories per minute and includes basketball, bicycling (12 miles per hour), jogging, racquetball, and swimming (moderate-to-fast pace). It is perhaps most useful to monitor the types of exercise performed and the amount of time spent exercising each day along with monitoring your food intake. This way you can determine how close you are to your goal of daily exercise.

- People use a variety of excuses for not exercising. These excuses include "I'm too tired"; "I have more important things to do"; "I don't feel good enough"; "It's no big deal if I miss one day." You can use "disputing responses" to dispute the logic of these excuses. For example, some disputing responses for "I am too busy" include "Exercise does take time. It takes time to invest in myself, my health, my well-being. I can make exercise a high priority in my life."

- Most middle-aged exercisers experience a variety of common injuries and illnesses. Flus, colds, and other illnesses can interfere with the momentum you develop as a consistent exerciser. Perhaps of greater concern are injuries like knee problems and back problems. It helps to expect and plan for such interferences to your exercise regimen. You can also take an aggressive approach to managing illnesses and injuries. For example, usually you can exercise a day or two before you think you can when recovering from a cold or a flu.

  Many injuries can lead to alternative forms of exercise, such as walking instead of jogging or swimming instead of playing racquetball. Athletic trainers, physical therapists, and chiropractors can provide some aggressive treatment for many common ailments. Try to pursue a medical approach that really makes sense to you and seems to help. Remember that the healing arts remain more art that science. If you keep this in mind and persist in investigating methods of healing injuries, you will learn to manage your weight even when your body becomes imperfect.

  The American Heart Association also suggests the following

helpful hints to avoid or prevent injuries: (1) stretch, warm up, and cool down; (2) build up your level of activity gradually; (3) listen to your body for early warning signs; (4) be aware of possible signs of heart problems; (5) take appropriate precautions for special weather conditions.

- It helps to keep your exercising in perspective. Becoming a consistent exerciser means becoming an exerciser who persists despite variations in the weather and changes in lifestyle. Consistent exercisers try a wide variety of activities. Walking can beget jogging. Health club memberships can beget playing racquetball or using trainers to assist in weight lifting.

# Epilogue

The following quotations are from "The Mind of a Marathoner," by William P. Morgan.

- "I perform complicated mathematical computations in my head (calculus) during a race."

- "Before a race, I actually pick out a series of CDs from my collection. I leave the CDs at home, but then I play the music from them during a race. Sometimes I 'groove on Beethoven' and sometimes I go 'mostly Mozart'."

- "I review my entire education, from first grade through my postdoc. I really like these recall sessions because I get to remember my favorite teachers, friends, and things I accomplished."

- "I like to stare at my shadow when I run. I find it fascinating to watch as my body leaves and enters the shadow from time to time and then seems to return back to me. I guess it's a 'Peter Pan' thing."

- "I design a house. Sometimes it is a Cape Cod, other times a Victorian. I complete the blueprints, dig a footing with a pick and shovel, pour the concrete, lay the blocks, put up the frame, then the roof, nail each shingle separately, wire the house, plumber it, plaster the walls, paint it inside and out, and then I do the interior decorating. I also landscape the yard, walk out onto the road and inspect my masterpiece."

- "I visualize the faces of two of my co-workers on the blacktop as I am running. I hate these people and I step on one face and then the other face the entire 26 miles!"

# 7

# Taking Control:
# Improving Self-Control

## Self Versus Other Control

Who controls you? In the table on the next page, assign a percentage of control either to yourself or to others for the behaviors listed. The total percentage assigned for each item should equal 100 percent.

Most people assign high percentages of control to themselves for several of these behaviors. You decide when to study, when to eat, and how to interact with others at parties. At least this applies to adults. For children, parents control a good deal more of eating, studying, and even talking. Other people and groups control you more regarding driving, behaviors in funeral parlors and libraries, and taxes, but you remain an active participant even in these circumstances. You could, for example, go to your nearest public library and start signing "Yesterday" or Barney's theme song. People would stare at you. Even if you rival Elvis, library staffers would soon ask you to stop singing. Yet you *could* begin singing even in that setting, if you decided to. You could also tell a joke anywhere, even at a funeral. Actually, some jokes get big laughs at funerals. Other jokes bomb at funerals, just like they do at bars.

Depending on the way you look at it, almost all of your behaviors are largely controlled by you. Control is not "on" or "off." Control is "more" or "less" in your hands. This chapter focuses on behaviors that most people view as controlled to a great degree by the individual.

## Five Phases of Self-Control

Self-control can be defined as the process by which you control your own behaviors in order to achieve desired goals. Self-control involves setting

## Control and Behavior

| Behaviors | You | Others |
|---|---|---|
| Eating | _____ | _____ |
| Smoking | _____ | _____ |
| Studying | _____ | _____ |
| Exercising | _____ | _____ |
| Talking with others at a party | _____ | _____ |
| Asking questions in a classroom | _____ | _____ |
| Telling jokes in a church | _____ | _____ |
| Singing in a library | _____ | _____ |
| Telling jokes in a funeral parlor | _____ | _____ |
| Telling jokes in a bar | _____ | _____ |
| Singing in a choir | _____ | _____ |
| Reading a magazine | _____ | _____ |
| Reading a street sign | _____ | _____ |
| Paying bills | _____ | _____ |
| Calling your mother | _____ | _____ |
| Paying your taxes | _____ | _____ |

goals and planning, observing, evaluating, rewarding, and punishing your own thoughts and actions. Psychologists have studied these processes for several decades. Research has focused on how people observe themselves and which types of goals help them change.

A very useful way to organize all of this information is to think of self-control as something that occurs in phases. The names of the five phases of self-control and the beliefs that characterize them are:

1. **Problem Identification:** Change is possible.

2. **Commitment:** Change is desirable.

3. **Execution:** Change is achievable.

4. **Environmental Management**: Change is promoted in supportive environments.

5. **Generalization:** Long-term change is possible.

## Problem Identification

Jack didn't see the problem. His doctor did. Jack came for a professional consultation only at his doctor's insistence. Jack weighed 550 pounds. He was 42 years old, lived with his parents, didn't work, couldn't fit behind the wheel of a car, had very limited connections with his friends, but, he insisted, "I don't really have a problem."

Jack's story is remarkably common. I've seen dozens of people who have adapted to life in this very unusual way. Food becomes their primary relationship. Food is always there when they need it. Food is dependable, interesting, and soothing. Unfortunately, relationships with food, when taken to great extremes, leave little room for much else. Jack didn't see that. Others like him similarly adapt to extreme levels of obesity in this peculiar way. They develop relationships with take-out restaurants. They preoccupy themselves with thoughts and types of food. They have collections of take-out menus that rival other people's collections of friends' names and numbers, stamps, coins, golf clubs, and flowers.

You can see how identifying something as a problem can become the biggest barrier to effective self-control. If Jack and others like him do

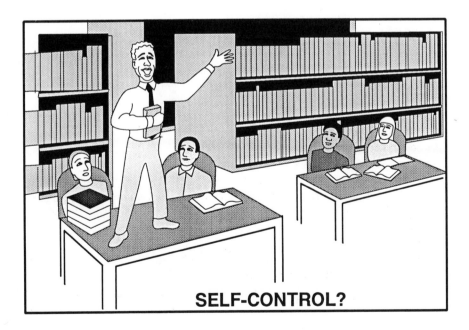

**SELF-CONTROL?**

not perceive their weight, eating patterns, or exercising patterns as problems, how can I (as a professional therapist) help them change? The answer is, I can only help them change if I can first help them identify problems.

Consider the following quotes from other people who had great difficulties defining weight control as a problem for themselves:

- "I like being big."

- "I never overeat."

- "I am a teacher. That's plenty of exercise!"

- "I don't have time for exercise in my life. I just have to control what I eat."

- "I can't be bothered with self-monitoring."

- "I can only eat what I really like. I only like really good food. Those no-fat products are awful."

Do these problems with "problem identification" sound familiar to you? You, like most readers of this book, are probably searching for solutions to a problem. This means that you already recognize some significant limitations in your eating and exercising patterns. However, perhaps you have children or a spouse who does not acknowledge problems when they really exist. Or perhaps you have significant difficulties in other aspects of your life. You get to go around this planet a grand total of *one time*. If you find yourself struggling with some issues, consider identifying those issues as problems.

You can help yourself and your friends and family identify problems by taking stock of what works and what doesn't work in your life. Are there any aspects of your life that clearly do not work? Do you enjoy the company of your friends and family? Do you feel satisfied with your job? Do you manage your money as effectively as you could? Consider all aspects of your life and ask yourself if they function the way you want them to right now. If you find far less than 100 percent satisfaction with job, family, friends, money, neighborhood, or any other issues, consider identifying those issues as problems. If you define something as a problem, you may be able to find a solution to it. If you fail to identify problems when problems really exist, your life will roll along in an unsatisfying way.

If you have family or friends with obvious weight control problems who seem reluctant to deal with them, what can you do? You can talk to them as you would like to talk to yourself. That is, you can help your friend or family member consider the consequences of failing to identify weight control as a problem. Perhaps you can discuss health concerns or social consequences. These discussions are tricky. People who adapt to obvious problems by denying their existence do not like to be confronted with the problems. Denial is a form of self-protection. If your family members or friends use denial, they will resist efforts to unmask that denial. Very genuine and gentle confrontations often produce good outcomes. It also helps to have specific recommendations in mind. Many weight controllers who have given up the struggle will argue, "I've tried everything and nothing helps!" This type of statement represents another form of denial. Persistence always produces positive outcomes. Giving up always produces negative outcomes. This is especially true for weight control. The biology of excess weight continues to create more difficulties as time goes by. Only through persistent efforts can weight controllers manage this biology reasonably well. Without persistent efforts, the biology takes over and the person becomes bigger and bigger.

Sometimes gentle confrontation helps people identify problems they have buried through denial. Other times, gentle confrontation gets nowhere. Discussion of the consequences of excess weight or alternative steps may not prove useful. More intensive and intrusive efforts sometimes work. For example, one of my client's sisters (Debbie) weighed more than 300 pounds. The weight and other aspects of Debbie's life did not work well for her. Yet she denied that she had any problems and lived a very unhappy existence. My client tried gentle confrontation and discussion. She sent Debbie articles about alternative approaches, as well. Debbie had given up. Her life was miserable, but she was afraid to try to change it.

My client gathered her family together and invited Debbie over. The entire family discussed Debbie's problems in a positive, supportive way. The family agreed to provide a variety of sources of support, including financial and emotional support. Debbie sought professional help within one week of this family meeting. If you don't feel comfortable doing something like this on your own, you could involve a professional therapist in such a confrontation. Many families couldn't get through this confrontation effectively on their own. A variety of mental health professionals could make it a constructive experience. If you want such assistance, seek out a family therapist in your area who comes highly recommended. Besides asking friends and co-workers to identify such individuals, you can inquire at local hospitals.

## Commitment

How committed are you to losing weight and increasing your exercising? The following "Commitment Questionnaire" will give you some idea. Read each item. If you see the word "BLANK" in the questionnaire, first substitute "exercise" and then substitute "weight loss." Then enter a number from 1 to 5 in the columns under "Exercise" and "Weight Loss" to describe your current feelings:

5 = Extremely characteristic of me

4 = Somewhat characteristic of me

3 = Neither characteristic nor uncharacteristic of me

2 = Somewhat uncharacteristic of me

1 = Extremely uncharacteristic of me

In this way, you can create a commitment score for both exercise and weight loss by totaling the ten items under each column.

# Commitment Questionnaire

| Items | Exercise | Weight Loss |
|---|---|---|
| 1. I'm very committed to BLANK. | _____ | _____ |
| 2. I'm really eager to develop the kind of self-discipline I need to BLANK. | _____ | _____ |
| 3. I'm good at keeping my promise to BLANK. | _____ | _____ |
| 4. When I find BLANK difficult, I try especially hard to stick with it. | _____ | _____ |
| 5. I will persist at BLANK despite pain and discomfort. | _____ | _____ |
| 6. Sometimes I push myself harder than I should when attempting to BLANK. | _____ | _____ |
| 7. I'm determined to reach my goals regarding BLANK. | _____ | _____ |
| 8. I've gathered a lot of willpower for BLANK. | _____ | _____ |
| 9. I will persist at BLANK despite occasional failures. | _____ | _____ |
| 10. I will not let myself down regarding BLANK. | _____ | _____ |
| **Totals** | _____ | _____ |

According to research on a related questionnaire conducted by Rod Dishman and his colleagues, you can interpret your scores as follows:

40 or more = High degree of commitment

35 - 39 = Moderate degree of commitment

34 or less = Low degree of commitment

Did you notice a difference in your degree of commitment to weight loss versus exercise? Many weight controllers report tremendous degrees of commitment to weight loss. Commitments to exercise rarely match commitments to weight loss. The previous chapter on exercise showed that persistent weight controllers' commitments to weight control match their commitments to exercise. How can you increase your commitment to exercise? You can recall the Decision Balance Sheet described in Chapter 2. Consider the following Decision Balance Sheet for exercise that one of my clients completed recently.

| Advantages of Exercising | Disadvantages of Exercising |
| --- | --- |
| Improved weight control | Hard to maintain |
| Improved muscle tone | Too many aches and pains |
| Feel better | Stressful fitting into schedule |
| Improved health | Some people have heart attacks while exercising |
| Take control over biology | Look silly, awkward while exercising |

If your commitment to exercising was less than your commitment to losing or controlling your weight, consider writing out your own Decision Balance Sheet with the advantages and disadvantages of exercising. After writing it out, sit back for a few minutes and look it over. Ask yourself, "Did I forget something?" You may wish to set the list aside for a few days and look it over again at some later point. It helps to add new items to both sides of it. The previous chapter on exercising describes dozens of advantages of exercising. You could use some of those items on your own list as well.

Another worthwhile device for improving commitment is to use disputing responses. An example of using this approach with exercise was presented in the previous chapter. You may also find it helpful to dispute other rationalizations about your weight control efforts. For example, if you find yourself thinking that you will focus on your eating tomorrow or next week, how can you dispute that?

You can discover yet another method for improving commitment by talking to friends and family members. When you make a commitment public, you increase your chances of working effectively to achieve it. Consider discussing your intentions to change over the next several months with your best friends or family members. These discussions can promote change because friends and family members will ask you about your efforts when they see you. This creates a positive pressure that helps many people improve their self-control.

Commitment involves setting goals. When you commit to change, you usually commit to change something specific. Hundreds of research studies have compared different types of goals. Which of the following types of goals do you think produce the best outcomes?

| Do Your Best Goals | Specific Goals |
|---|---|
| I will do my best to lose weight this month. | I will monitor all the food I eat and total calories consumed each day, every day this month. |
| I will really try to get myself together this week. | I will exercise for at least 30 minutes, at least three times each week during this month. |
| I will exercise a lot more this month. | I will talk to my husband about watching the kids for me during the mornings on the weekends so I can exercise for one hour on both Saturday and Sunday. |

The more specific goals usually produce much better effects than the "do your best" goals. Saying "I will do my best" amounts to saying very little. Talk is cheap. However, when talk includes measurable outcomes, it becomes a real motivator.

Do you think difficult or easy goals produce the greatest degree of self-controlled behavior change? Compare your reaction to the following types of goals:

| Easy Goals | Hard Goals |
|---|---|
| Exercise for at least 5 minutes twice a week for this month. | Exercise for at least 60 minutes at least five times per week. |
| Keep percent of fat consumed under 30 percent at least four days per week during this month. | Keep percent of fat consumed to 20 percent or less every day. |

The answer to this one is a little tricky. The answer is: It depends. Easy goals produce better outcomes when learning a difficult task or trying something new. More challenging goals produce better outcomes when tasks are very simple or very familiar. A novice at weight control and exercising may persist more effectively with relatively easy goals at first. More experienced weight controllers might benefit most from challenging, but realistic, goals.

One of my clients began exercising by setting a goal of 20 seconds a day using an exercycle at home. She gradually increased her goal to 45 minutes per day. She met every goal she set. She also lost more than 150 pounds and became an extremely effective exerciser. I have seen many other clients who set unrealistically difficult goals, such as "to keep percent of fat under 10 percent" or "to eat only dairy products, eggs, and vegetables forever." A few people perform beautifully after setting these stringent goals. Most, however, fail to meet their goals and then struggle to stay focused at all on the bigger goal of weight control.

You cannot use goals effectively unless you obtain feedback about your progress. Some people make New Year's resolutions to lose weight. Then they never take their scales out of their closets. Some students commit to studying longer and harder. Then some of these students fail to keep track of the number of hours they study per day or per week. They establish these goals in a vacuum of information about progress. Goals set without feedback produce no effects.

The three principles of goal setting just discussed have to do with the definition of goals, difficulty of goals, and use of feedback about progress toward goals. To summarize:

1.  *Define your goals clearly and specifically.* Clear goals are easily measured, such as the goal to exercise three times per week. Unclear goals are difficult to measure, such as "to do my best at increasing exercising."

2.  *Set easy goals when pursuing tasks that are very new or very difficult. Set moderately challenging or very challenging goals after experience with a task or when pursuing something very easy.* For example, experienced weight controllers usually eat modest amounts of high-fat foods. This makes goals such as "avoid high-fat foods" or "consume less than 30 percent of calories from fat at least three days per week" rather meaningless. If you already avoid high-fat foods, chances are it won't help you to set that very general, very easy goal. "To consume 20 percent of calories from fat at least five days per week," on the other hand, might challenge even rather experienced weight controllers.

3.  *Obtain frequent measures of progress toward goals.* You must measure the percent of calories consumed from fat if you wish to pursue goals about percent of fat consumed. In a similar way, when you monitor the frequency of your exercising, you make goals about frequency of exercising meaningful.

# Very Specific Plan

| Monday: | 6:00 A.M. | Wake up |
|---|---|---|
| | 6:30 A.M. | Walk 30 minutes |
| | 7–8:00 A.M. | Shower, get dressed, have breakfast Breakfast: Shredded wheat and skim milk, plus 1/2 banana |
| | 12:00 Noon | Lunch: Turkey sandwich on whole wheat bread, lettuce and tomato, mustard; one apple |
| | 3:00 P.M. | 15-minute walk |
| | 6:30 P.M. | Dinner: Chicken (3.5 oz), rice, broccoli, plus salad (low-calorie dressing) |
| | 8:30 P.M. | Snack: 3 cups air-popped popcorn |
| Tuesday: | 6:00 A.M. | Wake up |
| | 6:30 A.M. | Walk 30 minutes |
| | 7-8:00 A.M. | Shower, get dressed, have breakfast Breakfast: Shredded wheat and skim milk, plus 1/2 banana |
| | 12:00 Noon | Lunch: Turkey sandwich on whole wheat bread, lettuce and tomato, mustard; one apple |
| | 3:00 P.M. | 15-minute walk |
| | 6:30 P.M. | Dinner: Frozen low-calorie entree (300 calories or less), plus salad, plus orange |
| | 8:30 P.M. | Snack: 3 cups air-popped popcorn |
| Wednesday: | 6:00 A.M. | Wake up |
| | 6:30 A.M. | Walk 30 minutes |
| | 7–8:00 A.M. | Shower, get dressed, have breakfast Breakfast: Shredded wheat and skim milk, plus 1/2 banana |
| | 12:00 Noon | Lunch: Turkey sandwich on whole wheat bread, lettuce and tomato, mustard; one apple |
| | 3:00 P.M. | 15-minute walk |
| | 6:30 P.M. | Dinner: Vegetable soup plus salad |
| | 8:30 P.M. | Snack: 3 cups air-popped popcorn |

| Thursday: | 6:00 A.M. | Wake up |
|---|---|---|
| | 6:30 A.M. | Walk 30 minutes |
| | 7–8:00 A.M. | Shower, get dressed, have breakfast<br>Breakfast: Shredded wheat and skim milk, plus 1/2 banana |
| | 12:00 Noon | Lunch: Turkey sandwich on whole wheat bread, lettuce and tomato, mustard; one apple |
| | 3:00 P.M. | 15-minute walk |
| | 6:30 P.M. | Dinner: Chicken (3.5 oz), rice, broccoli, plus salad (low-calorie dressing) |
| | 8:30 P.M. | Snack: 3 cups air-popped popcorn |
| Friday: | 6:00 A.M. | Wake up |
| | 6:30 A.M. | Walk 30 minutes |
| | 7–8:00 A.M. | Shower, get dressed, have breakfast<br>Breakfast: Shredded wheat and skim milk, plus 1/2 banana |
| | 12:00 Noon | Lunch: Turkey sandwich on whole wheat bread, lettuce and tomato, mustard; one apple |
| | 3:00 P.M. | 15-minute walk |
| | 6:30 P.M. | Dinner: Frozen low-calorie entree (300 calories or less), plus salad, plus orange |
| | 8:30 P.M. | Snack: 3 cups air-popped popcorn |
| Saturday: | 6:00 A.M. | Wake up |
| | 6:30 A.M. | Walk 30 minutes |
| | 7–8:00 A.M. | Shower, get dressed, have breakfast<br>Breakfast: Shredded wheat and skim milk, plus 1/2 banana |
| | 12:00 Noon | Lunch: Turkey sandwich on whole wheat bread, lettuce and tomato, mustard; one apple |
| | 3:00 P.M. | 15-minute walk |
| | 6:30 P.M. | Dinner: Vegetable soup plus salad |
| | 8:30 P.M. | Snack: 3 cups air-popped popcorn |
| Sunday: | 6:00 A.M. | Wake up |
| | 6:30 A.M. | Walk 30 minutes |

| 7–8:00 A.M. | Shower, get dressed, have breakfast<br>Breakfast: Shredded wheat and skim milk,<br>plus 1/2 banana |
| 12:00 Noon | Lunch: Turkey sandwich on whole wheat<br>bread, lettuce and tomato, mustard; one<br>apple |
| 3:00 P.M. | 15-minute walk |
| 6:30 P.M. | Dinner: 1 1/2 cups pasta, low-calorie<br>tomato sauce (3/4 cup), plus salad |
| 8:30 P.M. | Snack: 3 cups air-popped popcorn |

## Execution

### Long-Term Planning

Let's say you establish a clearly defined, challenging, yet achievable goal for which you obtain adequate amounts of feedback. Now what? What is your plan? Plans are a proposed series of steps or subgoals that establish pathways to achieve goals. Some plans are very specific and detailed. Other plans are about as global as "do your best" goals. Consider the following two sets of plans and decide which would produce the best outcomes.

## Moderately Specific Plan

- Consume no more than 20 percent of total calories from fat this week.

- Exercise (walk, slow jog, Stairmaster at health club) a minimum of 20 minutes, at least six times this week.

- Eat no fried foods this week.

- Eat no desserts that include sugar as a primary ingredient this week.

- Use only air-popped popcorn, pretzels, and fruit for snacks all week.

- Self-monitor eating (including fat, percent of fat consumed each day) and exercising.

Which plan would work better for you? Many weight controllers think that highly specific plans are what they "need." Weight controllers have become used to reading and attempting to use specific diets. The very specific plan in the preceding example shows the obvious flaw of such dietary plans. Only a robot could live with such a stringent plan.

What happens if you decide to eat an apple when your plan calls only for air-popped popcorn? Do you feel guilty because you violated your plan? What if you sleep in on a Saturday morning? That ruins your plan as well. What if you get sick and tired of turkey sandwiches? When specific plans are violated, people often feel guilty and self-critical. These reactions lead to avoidance of the overall effort of effective weight control. The "baby gets thrown out with the bath water" when plans become too specific and rigid.

By contrast, the moderately specific plan allows for a reasonable (human) range of flexibility. It still meets the three criteria for effective goal setting: clear and specific, moderately challenging, and provides feedback. Yet people can live with such moderately specific plans. They provide direction and enhance commitment. They avoid promoting guilt because they are reasonable and flexible. By using moderately specific plans, you can protect yourself from feeling guilty about normal deviations from ideals. No one eats or exercises perfectly. At least no one does that forever. Effective weight control does not require perfection. It does, however, require consistent focusing. If you maintain an attitude of acceptance of your own reasonable deviations from perfection, you can maintain that critical focus. People in Tentative Acceptance or Lifestyle Change stages of change (as discussed in Chapter 3) really understand the importance of this kind of acceptance.

This moderately specific plan directs weight controllers toward a clear, challenging goal while allowing for the normal fluctuations of day-to-day life. It provides for various options. Weight controllers who adopt it could walk one day, jog the next, and even skip exercising altogether one day without violating the overall effort of persistence. Generally, then, moderately specific plans produce far better outcomes than highly specific, rigid plans.

Most plans cover relatively short periods of time. people often plan to exercise in a certain way for the next few days, weeks, or months. Similarly, you might plan dinners for one week or two weeks at a time. Some plans cover greater amounts of time. These often involve vacations or holidays. Such relatively long-term plans can cover several months and perhaps as much as a year. What about a lifetime plan? Do you have any long-term plans for your future? Perhaps you have such long-term plans regarding your family or your career. Consider the remarkable example of a long-term plan for a career written by B. F. Skinner more than 60 years ago. B. F. Skinner followed his plan amazingly well. Perhaps his plan helped him become one of the most influential psychologists in history.

> In a rather expansive mood, I drew up plans for the second thirty years of my life:
>
> November 17, 1932
>
> Plan of the Campaign for the Years 33-60

1. *Experimental Descriptions of Behavior. Continue along present lines. . . .* No surrender to the physiology of the central nervous system. Publish.

2. *Behaviorism vs. Psychology.* Support behavioristic methodology throughout. . . . Don't publish much.

3. *Theories of Knowledge (scientific only).* Definitions of concepts in terms of behavior . . . include a theory of meaning. Publish late.

4. *Theories of Knowledge (nonscientific).* Literary criticism. Behavioristic theory of creation. Publish very late if at all. These are in the order of importance, although 2 and 3 are about equal.

By far the greater bulk of time should go on 1.

Plan for the years 60–(?) (These are beyond my present control.)

(B. F. Skinner, *The Shaping of a Behaviorist*)

B. F. Skinner followed his long-term plan to a considerable degree. Perhaps his willingness to take such a perspective on his life contributed to his astounding productivity. Can you apply a similar perspective to your own weight control plan? This perspective calls for an analysis of what you will do, not next week, not next month, but for the next several years at least.

It may prove helpful to consider four steps of a long-term plan that I routinely recommend to people who inquire about how to lose weight. The plan includes a commitment to regular weigh-ins (at least once a week). It also assumes a strong commitment to making weight control a part of your life. Beyond that, the following four steps compose a lifetime plan for effective weight control:

1. Try self-directed change.

2. Increase involvement of family and friends.

3. Join a reasonable weight control program.

4. Join a long-term professional program.

**Step 1: Try self-directed change.** This phase of the plan includes making changes in eating and exercising patterns. It involves monitoring food intake and exercise expenditure. It also consists of taking whatever steps seem necessary to increase exercising. This could include developing a walking program or joining a health club. You should show meaningful results within a few months. Weight losses in the range of one-third to one pound per week seem reasonable.

**Step 2: Increase involvement of family and friends.** If step 1 does not produce positive results within several months, it's time to ask for help from others. Friends might consider beginning a walking program or playing racquetball on a regular basis. Your spouse might provide support in other ways. For example, your spouse could review self-monitoring records if you find it difficult to maintain them on your own. Beware of asking your spouse to help, however. Quite often spouses become too critical, which creates more tension and negativity than progress. Occasionally, they provide an appropriate level of positive support that can promote improved weight control.

**Step 3: Join a reasonable weight control program.** Two programs pass my test for "reasonableness." Both Take Off Pounds Sensibly (TOPS) and Weight Watchers provide good information at reasonable cost. They have both been around for more than 30 years. TOPS is a no-cost or minimal cost club that people join to support each other's weight control efforts. The groups vary in size and quality. The information TOPS provides seems accurate, although certainly not sophisticated. TOPS encourages members to monitor everything they eat and to weigh in at least once a week. Both of these encouragements can help improve weight control.

Weight Watchers, like TOPS, is widely available and provides strong encouragement for monitoring and weighing in regularly. Weight Watchers provides more up-to-date information and more formal presentations. Weight Watchers' meeting cost approximately $15 per week. Useful materials are provided, and discussions can help promote increased commitment. However, both Weight Watchers and Tops include many different kinds of participants. These approaches do not encourage individualized planning or attention. Many people drop out of these programs almost as quickly as they join them. On the other hand, many people benefit from these nonprofessionally conducted programs. If steps 1 and 2 produce inadequate progress, you might want to consider joining TOPS or Weight Watchers for a useful motivational boost.

None of the other widely available commercial weight control programs pass my "reasonableness" test. They seem most interested in the financial aspects of the weight control business. They may ask you to invest in their food products or their supplements (such as vitamins). These investments generally produce minimal returns.

**Step 4: Join a long-term professional program.** At several major medical centers and hospitals throughout the country, professionals conduct intensive weight control programs, such as the Optifast program mentioned in Chapter 5. Other programs are conducted by experts on behavior change who help people set goals and stay focused using a variety of techniques. These professionally conducted programs cost more than TOPS and Weight Watchers. However, many health insurance policies cover at least part of the cost of these programs. If you find that steps 1 through 3 produce inadequate results, and you are willing to invest further in this effort, try step 4.

To find a professional program where you live or work, call local colleges, universities, and hospitals. Ask for psychology departments and, within those departments, ask for programs specializing in weight control. It may prove useful to ask for psychologists with "cognitive-behavioral" orientations or backgrounds. Essentially, this step involves looking for a cognitive-behavior therapy program for weight control. Any program that lasts for only a few weeks or a couple of months is not worth pursuing. Programs like Optifast and others provide services for many months and even many years for those so inclined. That's what you need if you go to this step. If your local calls prove unsatisfactory, consider calling one of the following two national organizations for information about individuals who take a cognitive-behavioral approach to weight control and who live in your area: Association for Advancement of Behavior Therapy (212-279-7970) and American Psychological Association (202-336-5500).

### Positive Self-Monitoring

Setting goals and planning for changes in behavior can nudge those changes along only when you keep gathering information about that behavior. Regular weigh-ins provide some information. However, self-monitoring (observing and writing down all aspects of eating and exercising) provides far more useful and complete information. As discussed in Chapter 3, self-monitoring is critical to effective weight control. When people stop observing themselves carefully, they often stop persisting. This certainly applies to weight control.

You may have observed this in your own life when you "forgot" to get on a scale for a period of several months or stopped focusing on the quality of your eating and exercising. When you did this, what happened? Your biology usually takes over. The fat cells eagerly and hungrily gobble up additional calories and add weight. You can self-monitor in both positive and negative ways. However, you don't coldly and objectively gather information about yourself. When you gather information about your own behaviors, you usually evaluate the information as you gather it. For example, when learning a new sport, do you concentrate on your errors or your effective executions? What have you observed others doing in such situations? Do golfers frequently praise themselves and ignore their mistakes? Do tennis players frequently congratulate themselves when they serve well and ignore the serves that go into the net for double faults?

Usually people systematically focus far too much attention on their errors or failures. Unfortunately, this pattern of "negative self-monitoring" often worsens exactly those behaviors you wish to change.

Positive self-monitoring means systematically gathering information about target behaviors in a positive manner. This could include keeping track of or highlighting minisuccesses. Negative self-monitoring, by con-

trast, means systematically gathering information about poor performances. Negative self-monitoring includes focusing on minifailures or mistakes. Especially when tasks are new or difficult, positive self-monitoring
often improves performance.

Research has shown that golfers who kept track of only their good
shots improved the quality of their swings and lowered their scores.
Bowlers who kept track of the positive aspects of their shot-making improved their performances. For example, cne study by myself and some
colleagues included 60 relatively unskilled women bowlers (bowling average 123.7). These blowers received either no instructions (control) or
instructions from a professional bowler on the seven components of effective bowling. Some subjects received the instructions from the professional bowler and also instructions on positive self-monitoring. The Self-
Monitoring Sheet shows the instructions and sample record of positive
self-monitoring. Positive self-monitoring instructions asked subjects to review the seven components of effective bowling after finishing each
frame. In this condition, bowlers then recorded a number on a sheet of
paper only when they believed they had executed a particular component
well. Negative self-monitors, in contrast, recorded a number only when

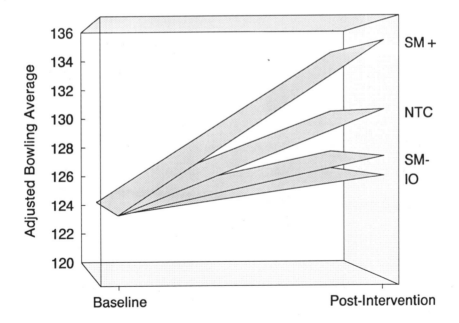

## Positive Self-Monitoring Helps Improve Performance

(SM+ means positive self-monitoring, SM- means negative self-monitoring, IO means information only, and NTC means no treatment control.)

## Self-Monitoring Sheet

### An example of instructions and a record-keeping form for positive self-monitoring in bowling

Name _____     Date _____

*Self-Instructions:* Before making your approach it is very important to remind yourself of the correct way to complete the final 3 components. Review in your mind the following: 1. Walk in a straight line for the approach. 2. Keep your elbow tight and locked on the push away, and use a straight pendulum-type swing that stays near your body. 3. At your finish position, your lead foot should be pointing toward your spot and you should be balanced at the line.

*Instructions:* After bowling each frame, review the seven components of Brian Power Bowling. For those components that you execute well, put a number from 1 to 3 in the space corresponding to that component: 1 = good; 2 = very good; 3 = excellent. If you do not do a good job on a particular component leave the box blank.

| Components | Frame 1 | Frame 2 | Frame 3 | Frame 4 | Frame 5 | Frame 6 | Frame 7 | Frame 8 | Frame 9 | Frame 10 |
|---|---|---|---|---|---|---|---|---|---|---|
| *Foot position:* same starting point each time | 3 | 3 | 3 | 3 | 3 | 3 | 3 | 3 | 3 | 3 |
| *Stance:* shoulders squared, elbow tucked into hip, knees relaxed | 2 | 3 | 3 | 2 | 3 | 2 | 2 | 2 | 3 | 3 |
| *Grip:* same grip for every shot, thumb and palm position correct | 2 | 3 | 3 | 2 | 2 | 3 |  | 1 | 3 | 3 |
| *Spot:* pick a spot and watch your ball roll over it. | 2 | 3 | 3 | 2 | 2 | 2 |  | 1 | 3 | 3 |
| *Approach:* take 2 to 3 seconds delay, walk in a straight line | 1 | 3 | 3 | 2 | 3 | 1 |  |  | 2 | 3 |
| *Push away:* elbow tight and locked, straight pendulum-type swing near body |  | 3 | 3 |  | 3 | 2 | 2 |  | 3 | 3 |
| *Finish position:* lead foot pointed toward spot, body balanced, square at the line | 2 | 3 | 3 |  | 3 |  | 2 |  | 3 | 3 |

Game Total 149

they believe they had executed a particular component poorly. The following graph shows that only the positive self-monitors significantly improved their bowling performance.

You can use the benefits of positive self-monitoring to improve your persistence at effective weight control. As you record information about your eating and exercising patterns, try to focus on what you did well. One method of doing this could involve using a highlighter to review each day's events. A well-controlled lunch or a good choice for a snack may deserve highlighting. Simply highlight, circle, or asterisk these more positive aspects of your daily eating and exercising records. Any exercising may deserve circling or highlighting. As you become a more effective exerciser, perhaps special notations about the quality of a particular workout would help. Even noting urges that you resisted effectively may prove useful. Consider the example below of a day's monitoring. This is a version of one of my client's records.

Notice that this client, Joe, focused on his exercising, breakfast, lunch, and resisting problematic urges. His other snacks, particularly popcorn, he felt, did not deserve special emphasis as positive events. This process of positively reviewing self-monitoring records does several important things. First, it encourages and reinforces self- monitoring. Second, it improves focusing. Not only did Joe self- monitor, he evaluated his own monitoring behavior. This is a way of enhancing his commitment and encouraging persistence. Finally, by staying positive, Joe avoided the natural tendency to become negative.

## Tuesday     (* = good control)

| | | Calories |
|---|---|---|
| *6:30 A.M. | Walked 3.6 miles | |
| *7:40 | Nutri-Grain wheat and raisins, skim milk | 220 |
| 10:00 | Bran muffin | 300 |
| *12:30 P.M. | Turkey on rye, lettuce, tomato, mustard | 320 |
| *2:30 | Resisted cookies at meeting | |
| 4:00 | Popcorn | 120 |
| 7:00 | Pasta, Healthy Choice tomato sauce, one piece of garlic bread | 650 |
| 8:00 | Apple | 90 |
| 10:00 | Popcorn | 200 |
| | **Total** | 1900 |

Many people who had a day like Joe's Tuesday might focus on the muffin that he ate at 10:00 A.M. or the fact that he had more snacks than he may have wanted to have that day. If Joe focused on such negative events, he might become upset with his efforts. Certainly, his efforts were admirable, although imperfect. They do not deserve abuse. Joe knows he ate the muffin and can attempt to avoid such foods the next day. If Joe were overly annoyed about such deviations from the ideal, this could lead to a downward spiral. Spirals often begin with negative self-monitoring and continue with decreased self-monitoring. This can lead to abandoning the effort at weight control.

Joe's example illustrates the importance of protecting yourself from your own negatives. Many of us are our own worst critics. This will not change simply by becoming aware of the tendency. Instead, most people benefit from using devices such as positive self-monitoring. These devices can protect you from your own self-critical nature.

### Mental Imagery

A world champion high-jumper, Dick Fosbury, spent several minutes on the runway "jumping in his head" before each of his jumps in competition. A world champion skier, Jean-Claude Killy, reported that his own preparation for one important race was to ski it mentally. An injury made it impossible for him to practice physically before that race. Killy claimed that the race turned out to be his best. Japanese gymnasts also use mental imagery regularly in their routines. For example, when attempting to learn the very difficult gymnastic skill called the iron cross, the Japanese gymnasts first think of contracting only those muscles needed to do the cross. Then they actually contract those muscles. Finally, they imagine themselves doing the iron cross. They try to visualize how they look and feel during the execution of the skill. In this way they learn how to relax muscles in their faces and necks that they do not want to contract when doing this particular move. This procedure may enable them to do very difficult strength moves while maintaining a totally relaxed expression on their faces.

With careful, consistent practice, you too can enjoy the benefits of mental imagery. You can use imagery to improve weight control by modifying patterns of eating and exercising. Terry Orlick, a well-known sport psychologist, provides some useful directions about how to use imagery to improve athletic performances. As you read the following instructions from his book, *In Pursuit of Excellence*, consider how you might apply it to your own exercising habits or your participation in sports.

It is probably best to start with very simple, familiar scenes and to gradually increase the complexity of the image. . .
Try to visualize the place where you usually work out.
Okay? Now, try to visualize the equipment you use to play

your sport (for example, ball, racquet, shoes, apparatus, etc.). If you are able to do this, try to see yourself doing very simple skills in your sport (running, passing, swinging, etc.). As this becomes easier, move into more complex skills. Keep in mind that the clearer and more complete the picture and the better you perform (or function) within that picture, the higher the probability of performing well ... in the real world. With practice, a scene can become very real just as dreams are very real.

If you experience problems calling up the image you would like, it sometimes helps to use a prop. For example, hold your hand out in front of you with fingers spread wide. Look at your hand for a few seconds, then immediately close your eyes and reproduce the image of your hand... This same process can be used to call up correct images of sports skills. You watch someone do the skill, close your eyes and replay it in your mind ... Vividness can be increased by really trying to put yourself into the gym or into the stadium. What do you see? What are you aware of? Are there people around? What is the surface like? Is it warm or cold?

Many of my clients use imagery to improve their commitments to exercise. They listen to weather reports and then, before going to sleep, they imagine themselves exercising in the morning. This imagery includes seeing themselves dressed appropriately for the weather conditions and waking up as soon as the alarm rings. Many clients lay out their exercise clothes the evening before. By using this "prop," they increase their commitment to "just do it."

The U.S. Olympic Committee provides some materials on the use of imagery for their athletes. Their materials discuss the use of imagery, guidelines for using imagery, and an analysis of the key components of imagery.

Some of the ways athletes can use imagery that weight controllers may also find helpful are to practice skills, overcome adversity, manage tension, and increase commitment.

**Rehearsing mentally.** You can use imagery to practice skills. Research indicates that once skills are reasonably well learned, athletes show improvements in performance by using imagery alone. Using imagery in sports or settings in which you have no experience will lead to little or no benefit. To improve performance by using imagery, you can put yourself into the sport or exercise situation in your mind. You can imagine yourself playing tennis or golf. Try to see your good shots and your mistakes. See if you can correct your mistakes and accentuate your better performances. Imagery serves as a blueprint to guide future performance and helps make skills more automatic.

**Preparing for competition.** Imagery can take you to a competition before the actual event. You can feel the excitement build and practice imagining yourself handling it as you would like to. You can also see yourself achieve the internal or mental state that has led to your best performances in the past. This could mean imagining yourself feeling relaxed but excited, ready to go.

An example of this preparation can apply to controlling food intake as well. Many people struggle with parties or celebrations in bars. If you are about to face such a challenge, imagine yourself in that situation before you actually get there. You could see yourself holding onto a glass of diet soda or bottled water. You can see yourself talking with people and using the social aspects of the situation as a focus. You might see chips, or peanuts, or appetizers pass in front of you. You can picture yourself handling those temptations very effectively and calmly.

**Overcoming adversity.** Athletes often experience surprising difficulties during competition. They may fail to make an easy shot or make an unforced error of some kind. Very strong negative or self-punitive reactions can magnify the problem. Have you seen athletes, or have you seen yourself, stomp around and curse in disgust after making a seemingly "stupid mistake." Such reactions often contribute to additional problems. Errors beget anger, which in turn begets more errors. This downward spiral can be prevented through imagery. Athletes can imagine themselves performing poorly in a critical moment and then rallying to regain their poise. Athletes can see themselves talking to themselves in an encouraging way, "It's a difficult game." "Stay calm, stay focused, and stay in the moment."

Weight controllers face many difficulties. For example, when working late, a group of people often order such readily available foods as pizza. The weight controller may find this high-fat food choice the only one available. By imagining yourself removing the cheese or more assertively managing the food order, you could help prevent this situation. Another image that proves useful sometimes is to imagine taking occasional lapses in stride. After eating pizza (unmodified in all its high-fat glory), consider using an image of someone who remains focused, writes down and calculates calories and fat grams, self-monitors the incident, and moves on from there.

**Managing tension.** Athletes often experience tension and pressure. They can calm down by imagining a favorite relaxing scene, such as a sunny day at the beach or a sunset in the mountains. You can use several relaxing scenes to help you feel mentally calm. You can call up these scenes when tensions run high. For example, at family functions or at work, imagery may help you cope with anger or anxiety. When you feel angry or frustrated, sit back in a chair in a quiet place and imagine a relaxing scene. You can use this technique to gain perspective and to remind yourself that alternatives other than food can help you get through difficult moments.

**Increasing commitment.** You can picture yourself fitting into clothes that you like and feeling more comfortable about your body. You can also imagine other benefits of weight control. Imagining increased self-esteem and self-confidence can add to your desire to achieve effective weight control. Just as athletes can imagine themselves winning, you can imagine yourself eating and exercising effectively and achieving your goals for weight control.

**How to use imagery.** The following are some guidelines on how to use imagery:

1. Create images in quiet, nondistracting environments. You can use imagery at almost any time: at home, at work, or before, during, and after exercising.

2. You may get the most out of your imagery if you relax yourself physically before concentrating on the imagery.

3. It helps to allow distracting thoughts and feelings to flow through your mind as you refocus on the image.

4. Within the image, use all your senses. It helps to imagine sights, feelings, and emotions within the image.

5. Use as vivid an image as possible.

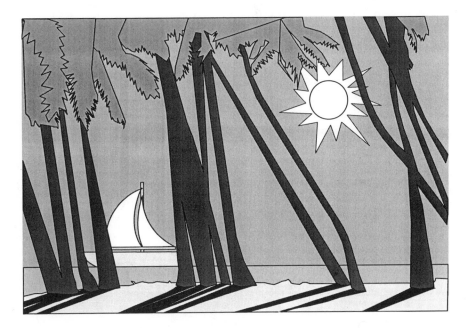

6. Start with easy images. Easy images are those with which you have the most experience.

7. As your skill at imaging increases, imagine yourself in more difficult and elaborate situations.

Key components of imagery are:

- **Sensory and emotional awareness.** You will struggle to create effective images if you do not know what the situation feels and looks like. This fact encourages you to attend carefully to your feelings and the visual aspects of your experiences whenever possible. One way of doing this is to ask yourself a series of questions in a variety of situations. For example, when in a bar or at a party, how can you describe typical experiences in these situations? What are the colors like? What are the people saying? What are the sound levels like? What are the smells like? To whom do you talk? What mood are you in?

- **Vividness.** Create images as rich in detail as possible. Use all of your senses, especially sight and touch. It takes time to create especially vivid images.

- **Controllability.** Images that you can control easily may produce better outcomes. If your image starts to become vague or distorted, stop and restart. Focus on yourself within the image. See yourself engaged in the situation completely from start to finish.

- **Perspective.** Some people use internal perspectives. They place themselves in the situation and see other people interacting with them as if they were there. Other people use images in which they function more like a television camera recording themselves within a context. Both internal and external perspectives can work very effectively. Try experimenting with images in which you do not see yourself in the image, but remain an active participant in the situation. Try that approach and replace it with one in which you observe yourself as if looking from the outside or from someone else's perspective.

- **Preparedness.** Imagery is not daydreaming. Imagery has a purpose. Before your imagery session, ask yourself, "What am I trying to do by using imagery now?" If you allow yourself to take imagery very casually, you will not reap maximum dividends from this technique. Instead, when you use imagery, place yourself in a relaxed state and spend several minutes concentrating. In this way, you can use this technique to sharpen your focusing and improve your commitment.

## Environmental Management

### Stimulus Control

Stimulus control refers to the ability of certain situations or stimuli to control patterns of behavior. This means that certain situations or stimuli can affect eating or exercising patterns in a direction that is either positive or negative. For example, when you see a commercial on television for fast-food hamburgers, you may feel particularly hungry and head toward the refrigerator. This means that watching TV can become a stimulus for eating.

Another example of stimulus control is the way the place where you eat can affect the likelihood of eating. People who eat while driving around in a car or in a bus are more likely to eat in many different situations than people who eat only in their kitchens or dining rooms. Some people eat when they are preparing food. For these individuals, the stimulus of preparing food affects their eating. Another example is the clock. When the clock strikes twelve, many people experience a strong desire to eat. The features of the environment such as the time of day, other people eating, food advertisements, and even the sight of food often affect overweight people more than non-overweight people.

The following suggestions use the principle of stimulus control to reduce the number of stimuli associated with problematic eating:

- **Decrease eating situations.** Attempt to limit the number of situations in which you allow yourself to eat. Try to focus your eating primarily in kitchens, dining rooms, and restaurants. Avoid eating in family rooms, living rooms, or while watching television. Also be aware that eating at your desk or while working at a computer can create stimulus control problems.

- **Place food only in food areas.** It is best to keep all the food in your house in food areas. Having food available in candy dishes or glove compartments of cars just causes more interest in eating than you need. If you avoid keeping or bringing food to your room for nighttime eating and snacking, you will also feel less hungry.

- **Discontinue non-eating activities in food areas.** In food areas such as kitchens and dining rooms, it would be most helpful if you primarily store, prepare, or eat food. Sometimes people work or sew or talk while sitting around kitchen or dining room tables. Try to avoid placing yourself in those situations. Food areas are associated with eating. If you put yourself in those areas frequently, you will stimulate your appetite. This makes it more difficult to avoid eating at times when you are trying to do other things.

- **Make eating a "pure experience."** Besides storing all food in one area and excluding non-eating activities from that area, it is helpful to make eating a pure experience. In other words, it may help you reduce the amount that you eat if you engage in no other activity other than consuming food while you eat. For instance, try to avoid watching TV, listening to the radio, reading newspapers, or working on school work while you are eating. You may, of course, talk with family or friends while eating, but try to avoid staying at the table after you finish eating. While you are eating, try to concentrate as much as possible on the taste, texture, and smell of the food. You may find that you enjoy eating more by focusing on the pure experience of eating rather

## Case History: Keeping Home Sweet Home Safe

Marge and her husband Mike have an excellent relationship. They work and play together and have a wonderful baby girl. They are both successful professionals, and they respect each other's abilities and talents.

Marge has a substantial weight problem. She began the program with me several years ago. At that time she weighed 220 pounds (she is 5-feet-2-inches tall). She locked into a remarkably long Honeymoon stage and lost weight very steadily for more than a year. She exercised fanatically and added weight training to treadmill, Stairmaster, and walking as her primary exercises. She relied on frozen foods, pasta, and potatoes as her mainstays. After about 1 1/2 years, she reached her weight goal (140 pounds). She diligently monitored all her food intake and her exercise output. Marge handled a variety of tensions effectively and received a lot of support from Mike. While she was in the Honeymoon stage, nothing Mike did or ate had any real effect on her. Unfortunately, Honeymoon stages do not last forever. Marge had some major conflicts at work, had to change jobs in a difficult situation, and her eating and exercising became less of a priority in her life. She began regaining weight and getting into binge eating occasionally. During this Frustration stage, Mike's eating habits began to have negative effects on Marge. Mike never had a weight problem and could eat almost anything he wanted to without gaining weight. He frequently ate potato chips, M&M's, and a variety of high-fat foods. When he and Marge watched the news or a movie at night, instead of munching on air-popped popcorn (as she did consistently during the Honeymoon stage), Marge began nibbling on Mike's high-calorie snacks. When she opened that door, she found it hard to close. In other words, once she began eating potato chips instead of air-popped popcorn, the popcorn seemed like "cardboard," and she found the higher-fat snacks "almost irresistible."

I encouraged Marge to bring Mike in for a meeting with me. The three of us discussed how Marge's problem was like a chronic disease. If Marge had a heart condition, cancer, or diabetes, Mike would have no problem making some adjustments in his life to keep Marge healthy. He had more trouble with this issue because he felt, "Don't I have a right to eat the way I want to?" We discussed this concern and concluded that Mike's freedom required some modification to help his wife stay healthy. He agreed to accommodate Marge and to keep all high-fat snacks out of the house. Marge found that it made it much easier for her to exhibit self-control when her environment was well controlled. Her Frustration stage passed into a Tentative Acceptance stage. She no longer snacked on high-fat foods, and she began getting back to her goal weight. During the past year or so, she has maintained a very good weight for her (approximately 150 pounds).

than on all the other activities associated with eating. For people who live alone, eating with less or different kinds of stimulation can make eating a pure experience. Many people who live alone eat while watching television or reading. Try eating without television if you live alone. Perhaps you will notice less "mindless" eating if you do this.

The story of Marge and Mike raises some important points. People sometimes think that good self-control means being able to stare at a chocolate cake five inches from your face and resist eating it for two hours. A much better form of self-control involves keeping the chocolate cake away from your face. In other words, self-control includes managing one's environment to promote healthy behaviors. Marge learned that her self-control was dependent on keeping her home safe. For Marge, a safe home was one in which no high-fat snacks were available. This applies to most weight controllers. It requires some adjustment by families of weight controllers to live like this. High-fat snacks do not help anyone have a better life. However, our culture encourages consumption of these foods. Some people feel deprived and angry if they cannot have them. Weight controllers are faced with the difficult task of convincing their families to help them take care of themselves by keeping these foods away from their homes. Remember, weight controllers have as much as 500 times greater biological responses to the sight, and perhaps even the thought, of some of these very tempting foods. Is it fair or reasonable for families of individuals who have this biological handicap to challenge this handicap on a daily basis? Instead, families can accommodate their weight controllers by eating high-fat foods outside of the home. Is that too much to ask?

The best way for weight controllers to encourage their family to make this transition is to take an understanding approach. Some weight controllers get into difficulties when they insist on changing their family's eating patterns overnight. They might say to their family, "It's time for us to get rid of all this junk food!" That approach encourages resentment and anger. An alternative would be to ask family members to understand the biological challenge faced by weight controllers. People respond much more favorably when they are asked to help rather than coerced to change. Consider using something like the following approach to make your home a safe home: "I really need your help. My biology responds very dramatically to the sight and smell of foods that are high in fat and calories. This makes it much more difficult for me to control my eating. If I have trouble controlling my eating, I don't feel good and I won't stay healthy and satisfied with myself. Because of this, I would like you to help me keep certain kinds of food out of the house. I know this is a sacrifice for you, and I would really appreciate it if you would do it for me." The exact wording makes no difference. The approach of asking for help, rather than demanding it, however, can make all of the difference. When cookies or potato chips "magically" appear, try a gentle reminder about your need for help.

## Generalization

The following are some personal experiences of three weight controllers who lost considerable amounts of weight and then relapsed.

> I had lost 42 pounds. It was quite a struggle. It took me almost a year of hard labor. Then there was this doughnut! I had been feeling so good, getting into some old clothes, and I just ate this doughnut. I figured, "I've got this thing controlled. I can eat a doughnut." The doughnut led to other foods like doughnuts. I started eating ice cream again. For some reason, I stopped exercising. It took me almost a year to lose the 42 pounds, but only a couple of months to regain it all, and then some.

> I joined the Optifast program. I ate nothing but the powder for 12 weeks and lost almost 50 pounds. I exercised practically every day (mainly walking). I kept participating in maintenance groups for 3 1/2 months after the initial fast. I lost another 5 to 10 pounds during that period. My relationship with my husband was never the greatest. We started having more bitter fights toward the end of the fast. Sometimes we would fight and scream at each other and other times we would be walking around each other in stony silence. We separated about the same time I discontinued participating in the maintenance groups in the Optifast program. Food became a reliable source of comfort

again. Instead of watching every fat gram I ate, I just let myself eat what I felt like eating. It didn't take long to regain the weight.

I joined a professional weight control program two years ago. I was a fanatic. I ate between 600 and 800 calories a day and exercised every day. I had to start out slowly because I was 120 pounds overweight. I started walking and then I graduated to fast walking and weight training. I bought a treadmill and a Stairmaster and turned my den into a minigym. I was determined to beat this thing! Somehow I managed to stay on this intensely focused program for over a year. I lost 110 pounds and was feeling really good. Then I broke my leg in a skiing accident. It was a hairline fracture, but it was enough to sideline my exercising for two months. I was frustrated and began losing focus. I discontinued my involvement in the program and stopped monitoring my eating and exercising. After the two months was over, I tried getting myself to walk again. It was painful and I had trouble staying with it. It would have been helpful for me to rejoin my program. I finally did that last week after regaining 95 of the 110 pounds that I had lost. It's painful to face myself. I tried making it on my own and I couldn't do it. I know I can get back into this again, and this time I'm never going to quit it.

The challenges of maintaining weight losses sometimes exceed those faced during weight loss. At least when you are losing weight, you can see clear signs of progress on a regular basis. After weight loss is achieved, the thrill of feeling in control, wearing smaller size clothes, and getting compliments gradually declines. (To some people, compliments are less than thrilling anyway.) Also, consider the nature of the goals for maintaining weight losses. The goals are rather vague and unclear. In contrast, goals for weight loss are specific and easily measured. Maintenance clearly provides less drama than weight loss, and the goals for maintenance are fuzzier than those for weight loss.

To maintain weight losses successfully, you must generalize, or transfer the skills you used to lose weight to new situations over long periods of time. Self-monitoring, low-fat eating, and frequent exercising must become part of your life. This "generalization phase" is extremely challenging. Many people find it very difficult to maintain the focus necessary for success over long periods of time. Think of weight loss as a challenge similar to driving a car in heavy traffic in a big city. You stay alert under these driving conditions because so much comes right at you. You have little change of losing focus on the traffic or your destination. However, when you get onto a major highway after coming out of the city, alertness

comes less naturally. The miles roll on and the traffic presents few challenges. The generalization phase resembles highway driving. Generalization, like alertness when driving on highways, demands focusing from
within. Weight loss, like driving in congested city traffic, involves responding to more immediate challenges with very clear feedback for mistakes.

Research and experience suggest a variety of ideas, techniques, and
issues that affect generalization of self-control for weight controllers,
which are discussed in the following sections.

### Lapse Versus Relapse

The biology of excess weight makes it *impossible for anyone* to eat
perfectly. Those hungry fat cells and associated hormones make an occasional french fry or doughnut virtually irresistible. Some studies show
that overweight people respond biologically as much as 500 times greater
than non-overweight people to the sight and even the thought of food.
Since perfection in eating is impossible, occasional lapses occur for even
the most persistent weight controller.

A *lapse* is a temporary problem; it is a temporary deviation from
the overall plan. Lapsing does not have to lead to relapsing. A relapse is
a full-blown change back into old, problematic styles of behaving.

Successful weight controllers persist in the face of the inevitable
lapses. They realize that an occasional doughnut or ice cream cone is simply a problem, not a catastrophe. They view these deviations as acceptable, not earthshaking. Lapses become relapses when you discontinue
monitoring of your eating and exercising. If you eat four pieces of pizza
and consider it a disaster, you may give up monitoring for that day, for
that week, or for that year. If you eat the pizza and consider it a problem
to be solved, you will write it down, calculate its calories, and try to understand how you could have presented that problem from occurring.

Consider the lessons in the following story about lapsing, told by
one of my most successful clients, Nancy.

> I went on vacation to Mexico and it was as if I had never
> heard of weight control. I just ate what I felt like, lay
> around in the sun, and had a great time. Maybe it was
> being in a different country where everything was different.
> Somehow I just forgot who I was and what my body was
> about.
>
> I came back after two relaxing weeks and stared at
> that metal monster in my bathroom. It took me two days to
> get back on it, but finally I did. I had gained eight pounds!
> I couldn't believe it. It's just not fair. It took me a while,
> but I realized that no one promised me that life was fair. I
> remembered what I had learned about the biological aspects
> of weight problems. I realized that my fat cells "never go
> on vacation." That's not fair, that's just the way it is.

I got back into monitoring my eating, and I got back out there and started walking every day again. The weight started to come back down. It took me two months to get back to where I was before that vacation. I'm hoping the lesson in this is to find a way of relaxing without ignoring what my body is about.

Nancy prevented her rather major lapse from becoming a full-blown relapse. More minor and usual lapses occur when people eat occasional high-fat or high-sugar foods. To prevent lapses from turning into relapses, remember two things:

- Lapses are inevitable.

- Lapses won't become relapses if self-monitoring is maintained.

After you experience the inevitable lapse, try to write it down and deal with it as a problem to be solved. Figure out what led to the lapse, forgive yourself for lapsing, and move on from there.

### Management of Injuries and Illnesses

Momentum is a magical thing. In weight control, as in many other aspects of life, you build momentum for change. You get into routines and rely on these routines to keep you going. Twisted ankles, back problems, flus, colds, and other problems can interfere substantially with momentum in weight control.

Aggressive management of injuries and illnesses can preserve some of the momentum for effective weight control. For example, one of my clients, David, developed chronic sinus infections after the birth of his second child. Children bring a lot of joy into life—but a lot of colds as well. David had allergy problems, but his children's "gift" of frequent colds increased his problems. Sinus infections are like mild colds that also produce fevers and sluggishness. Unfortunately, they don't go away in seven days. They tend to stick around for weeks if untreated by antibiotics. David found it difficult to maintain his jogging program, and thereby control his weight, because of these sinus infections.

He went to see an ear, nose, and throat specialist and an allergist. After a variety of tests, David and his doctors decided the best course of action for him was to begin using very strong doses of antibiotics. He was to take this medicine as soon as he felt a new sinus infection beginning.

Last year, David got his usual dose of four or five sinus infections. But, unlike the previous year in which these infections greatly interfered with his life, this year each time an infection began, the antibiotics let him feel pretty good after just two days. So this year he was incapacitated for approximately eight to ten days instead of the eight to ten weeks in the previous year.

Other clients like David pursue alternative exercises when illness, sprained ankles, or back problems interfere with their usual routines. Exercycling puts a lot less pressure on backs, and sometimes less on knees, than walking or running. These are challenging transitions, but also inevitable. Successful weight controllers become, essentially, middle-aged athletes. Athletes push their bodies hard. Weight controllers push their bodies hard, as well.

Many times, physicians and other specialists can help. But these helpers can also be quite frustrating. They offer solutions that sometimes don't work. Some solutions produce side effects that are worse than the problem. Searching for effective solutions might involve going from one health care professional to another until you find the right approach. Knee and back problems are notorious for this kind of frustration. Sometimes can help; sometimes physical therapists can help; sometimes orthopedic surgeons can help; and sometimes chiropractors can help. Persistent weight controllers keep trying until they find something that works. They also accept frustration as one of the more unpleasant results of doing what has to be done to remain successful.

In sum, the keys to effective management of injuries and illnesses are to:

- Be aggressive about seeking help when needed.

- Expect frustration when seeking help.

- Find alternative means of exercising as soon as possible when injuries or illnesses interfere with your usual routines.

### Scale Phobia

"I didn't want to get on a scale this week because I think I gained weight." Does this sound familiar? It's a problematic attitude that can lead to relapsing. Scales provide necessary information to weight controllers. If you avoid getting on a scale because you think you may have gained weight, you begin a pattern of avoiding self-monitoring. Remember, when people discontinue self-monitoring, they often discontinue effective self-control. Scales do not make judgments; only people can judge themselves. If you see a number that is higher than you like, you can do something about it. Avoiding the number on the scale just reinforces avoidance of the problem. If you avoid this problem, it never goes away. Your biology takes no vacations and cuts you no slack. You can try to make a deal with your biology, for example, "If I don't look at the consequences of what you do to me, will you be kinder and gentler toward me?" Your fat cells would answer, "No way! I just want to get filled up. I don't care when or how or what it takes to get me filled up. I just want fat."

The best way to kill a scale phobia is to get on the scale. You can simply commit to weighing yourself at least once a week and dealing with whatever number you see. A very large study conducted by Weight Watchers showed that people who maintain their weight successfully for one year or more used a three-pound window. That is, successful weight controllers in the Weight Watchers program observed their weights carefully. When they noticed that they had gained as much as three pounds, they aggressively focused on their eating and exercising again to bring the weight back down immediately. Their less successful counterparts, people who regained substantial amounts of weight within a year after losing it, used a ten-pound window. These individuals paid much less attention to their scales (weights). They allowed their weights to fluctuate by as much as ten pounds. They obviously had a more difficult time bringing their weights back down to acceptable levels after they had gained as much as ten pounds.

It helps to use a narrow weight window and to continue weighing yourself regularly every week. You might find it useful to keep a graph of your weight. Perhaps you could hang it on the inside of your closet. You can write down the date you weighed yourself and your weight. You can look at this graph every day when you're getting your clothes and think about what it means.

### Permanent Vacations

Most people find vacations relaxing, distracting, and enjoyable. Vacations are also dangerous to weight controllers. Vacations interfere with momentum. Vacations, like illnesses and injuries, cause changes in your usual routines. One of my clients, Renee, said, "I get into a 'vacation mentality.' The vacation mentality allows me to relax my restraint. I take it easy on myself. I don't force myself to exercise or count calories. I focus on my family and have fun." You can see that a "vacation mentality" can become a dangerous thing. Vacations can lead to decreases in exercise and reemergences of higher-fat, higher-sugar eating. Once these patterns reemerge, they are hard to break again.

People in the Lifestyle Change stage find a way of treating a vacation as an opportunity for increased exercise and a vacation from their own refrigerators and cupboards. That is, these individuals seek out exercise whenever possible during vacations, and they know it will be easier to resist snacking. In fact, people in the Lifestyle Change stage usually lose weight on vacations. They stay "aggressively self-protective" and find vacations the perfect opportunity to take good care of themselves. Vacations do not have to mean overindulgence. Relaxation and fun can occur without high-fat, high-sugar eating and sedentary living.

### Changes in Key Relationships

Major conflicts in key relationships can interfere with your life more dramatically than almost anything else. Can you recall what happened to you the last time you had a major conflict at work? Most people report

trouble sleeping and tremendous preoccupation when such conflicts occur. Conflicts at home produce even more dramatic symptoms. Major
lapses can quickly become relapses during periods of conflict with
friends, co-workers, and loved ones. The sense of "nothing else matters"
can make effective eating and exercising seem absolutely trivial during
these difficult times.

People almost always survive major conflicts with people who are
very important to them. When these conflicts occur, your very survival
seems threatened. Yet conflicts are very much a part of life. Millions of
people have divorced and had huge upheavals in their jobs. Yet they all
survive. Survival tactics include obtaining support from other friends during these difficult times. Exercise can serve as a meaningful outlet for
some of the tension that accrues. Eating high-fat and high-sugar foods
may only add to increased feelings of tension. Some weight controllers
find it helpful to join Weight Watchers or a professional program during
extreme periods of stress, such as those involving conflicts in relationships. These supportive steps can help weight control remain a priority.

To summarize, you can keep your focus on weight control strong during conflicts in key relationships if you remember that "this too shall pass";
seek support from friends and/or through programs that focus on weight
control; and use exercise and controlled eating as a means of coping.

### Work or Financial Crises

Losing a job or suffering major financial problems can interfere very
substantially with persistent weight control. These crises, like crises in
personal relationships, can make weight control seem trivial or unimportant. I've heard many clients say things like, "How can I worry about
the number of fat grams I eat when my world is crumbling around me?"
Part of the answer to this question lies in the value of exercising regularly
and low-fat/low-sugar eating. Weight control certainly takes effort and
focusing. Yet exercising effectively and eating in accord with a reasonable
plan produces important benefits in your mood and feelings about yourself. Weight control does not merely burden without benefit. During a
crisis on the job or a financial crisis, you can use weight control to provide
stability and support in your life. If you view it this way, you may keep
your exercising and eating patterns more effective than if you view
weight control as a burden without any payoff. How can it really help
you during a crisis to give up a pattern of eating and exercising that has
proved comfortable and satisfying in so many ways? Certainly eating
foods that are high in sugar provides some immediate tranquilizing effects. This is part of what draws people to candy bars and other "goodies"
during difficult times. Also, it may relieve some biological stress to decrease exercising or to relax your usual restraints about style of eating
during such crises. However, increased weight and increased guilt may
make such major lapses hardly worth their temporary benefits.

Consider working as aggressively as possible to solve both work and financial problems when they occur. Get help from friends and advisers about these situations. Begin a networking process to find another job, or take other steps to improve the job situation you are in. Remember that you are not on a diet. Your eating and exercising plan has become part of your life. Why give up an important and healthful part of your life just because another part of your life has gone awry? Consider finding alternative means of handling the stress, such as those emphasized in the next chapter, "Stress and Coping."

Robert Colvin and Susan Olson conducted a series of studies on 54 men and women who had lost at least 20 percent of their initial weights and maintained those losses for at least two years. Among the women they studied, average weight losses were over 50 pounds and had been maintained for more than six years. In their most recent report, one woman had regained 18 pounds from her original weight loss. This woman indicated that one of her two small businesses had failed, causing serious financial problems. Her son dropped out of college and returned to live at home. At about the same time, her elderly mother moved in from New York. As she was adjusting to this, her best friend's family was killed in an automobile accident.

This situation illustrates how disruptions in key relationships, financial and work crises, and other aspects in life can lead to problems, even for highly successful weight controllers. On the other hand, Colvin and Olson noted that virtually all their other "winners" maintained stable weights despite many strains: "subjects listed divorce, major surgery, death in the immediate family, and loss of home and possessions through fire as life events" that they coped with successfully, without regaining substantial amounts of weight (1984, *Addictive Behaviors*).

### Major Changes in Eating Environments

The following two stories show how major changes in environment can affect your eating patterns dramatically.

**Arnie:** "I got promoted a few months ago. I was really excited. It was a great opportunity. Unfortunately, it involved traveling two to three days per week. I figured, 'no big deal. I can handle this.' I didn't realize how much traveling around the country disrupted my usual routines. I found myself frustrated and irritated more of the time. Relaxation and cooling out time became less and less. I felt tired in the morning and found it difficult to exercise at my usual time. I wound up in meetings in which all kinds of food (like muffins, doughnuts, pizza, cheese, and crackers) were carted in during all hours of the day and night. My eating and exercising habits began to break down, and I began gaining weight."

**Jane:** "I got a divorce last year. The time before the divorce was the real struggle (for about two years). The divorce was a tremendous relief for me. My weight was reasonably stable during the years before the divorce. I couldn't believe it, but I gained 20 pounds during this past year. It was such an adjustment. All of a sudden, for the first time in almost ten years, I was living by myself. I thought that would make it so much easier to control my food. I didn't realize that being in an unhappy relationship in some ways created fewer temptations for me than being alone. I found myself feeling lonely. Other times, I went out with friends to dinners and parties—far more often than I had in the last ten years. I was drinking some more and eating bar food. I had more trouble sleeping, and that made it harder to get up early and exercise. I guess that's what did it."

Previous chapters discussed the difficulties associated with traveling. Traveling obviously creates many challenges for weight controllers. Any substantial modification in your living situation also creates problems to be solved. Moving out of your house and into a college dormitory, or moving out of a dormitory into an apartment, are transitions with which many of you are familiar.

If you recall those transitions in your own life, consider the impact they had on your eating and exercising. Have you ever heard of the "Freshman 10?" Many college freshmen report gaining ten pounds when they move into a college dormitory for the first time. These weight gains, while not well documented scientifically, may occur for some people because of the tremendous changes in their usual routines.

If you experience such disruptions in your life, the keys are to keep monitoring your weight and eating and exercising patterns; and if your weight and eating and exercising patterns begin to change in a problematic direction, take some steps to fix the problems. The latter point may include getting involved in a self-help or professional program, or it may include joining a health club. If you stay focused enough on this issue to observe the patterns of change in your eating, exercising, and weight, you put yourself in a position to handle changes effectively.

### Direct Versus Indirect Problem Solving

Susan Kayman and her associates conducted a study in which they compared "maintainers" to "regainers." Maintainers were formerly obese women who had lost at least 20 pounds and maintained that loss for at least two years. Regainers were obese women who regained weight after losing at least 20 pounds. The chart shows that the regainers used "escape-avoidance" methods of solving problems much more than maintainers. These methods include eating, drinking, smoking, sleeping, and wishing the problems would just go away as methods of coping. Regainers also failed to get as much support from others ("social support") as the maintainers. Most dramatically, maintainers reported confronting problems directly and aggressively—approximately ten times more frequently than regainers. Successful weight controllers in this study, and more gen-

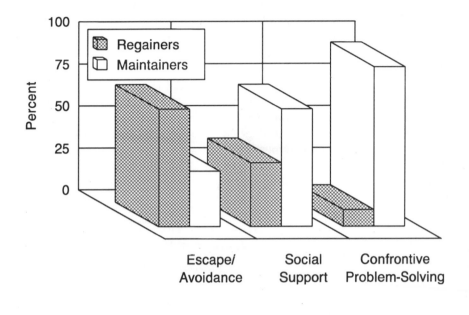

**Coping with Problems**

erally, seem to identify their problems relatively quickly and take steps to change as soon as possible.

### Abstinence Violation Effect (AVE)

Alan Marlatt and Judith Gordon identified a type of distortion in thinking that creates problems. The abstinence violation effect, or AVE, first involves making a commitment to "abstinence." Many people who change their habits (for example, people who quit smoking or alcohol, as well as successful weight controllers) make a commitment to abstain forever from a certain pattern of eating or drinking. Weight controllers who do this may view themselves as "dieters." What happens when a dieter eats a food that is not on the diet? For example, what happens when a dieter eats a piece of birthday cake? This dieter may view this initial lapse as a major conflict. The conflict might sound something like this in the head of the dieter, "How can I be a dieter if I ate a piece of birthday cake?" One way of resolving this conflict is to abandon dieting. In other words, abstinence violation effects are relapses that occur to reduce the conflict created by lapses. When weight controllers commit to unrealistically stringent standards for eating or exercising, they set the stage for AVEs. Following this commitment, initial lapses can produce major conflicts. These internal conflicts can be resolved by going into a full-blown relapse: "I can eat pizza and cookies now because I am no longer on a diet."

You can avoid AVEs by adopting more realistic and reasonable goals. It makes no sense to commit to abstinence for weight controllers. Weight controllers simply cannot control their biologies and their situations perfectly. If you commit to abstaining from all sugar forever, you set yourself up for an AVE. How can you handle the initial lapse, the first ice cream cone or piece of cake, when you adopt such an unreasonable goal? It is critical to avoid placing yourself in such a conflict. Instead, it helps to understand that weight controllers, even the most successful weight controllers, eat and exercise imperfectly. Lapses are inevitable. If you eat a problematic food, identify it as a lapse, write it down, and realize that a lapse, or two lapses, or a thousand lapses do not make you any less of a weight controller. You are an effective weight controller as long as you confront the issues involved with managing weight consistently and directly. You become a "non-dieter" or "non-weight controller" only when you stick your head in the proverbial sand. When you refuse to get back on a scale or discontinue observing your eating and exercising, then and only then do you become a non-weight controller.

### Healthy Obsession

When consistent exercisers stop exercising, even for one day, they get rather testy. Research has established that regular exercising is a positive obsession or addiction. That means that people get used to the feelings associated with exercising and rely on it to help them feel good. That same healthy obsession applies to persistent weight controllers. When weight controllers who are in the Lifestyle Change or sometimes Tentative Acceptance stages find their usual routines about eating, exercising, and monitoring disrupted, they also get testy. These individuals have developed a healthy obsession with weight control. They rely on a certain approach to eating and exercising and observing themselves in order to feel comfortable. Disruptions are greeted with annoyance, irritability, and dissatisfaction. This is the state you want to be in if you want to become a successful, persistent weight controller. You "want" to feel annoyed and irritable when something disrupts your usual routines. That reaction shows a very strong commitment to permanent weight control.

Some weight controllers become secretly happy when opportunities to stray from their usual patterns emerge. You may have noticed this in yourself or in others. "Oh well, I was at a party and there was nothing else to eat—so I ate!" Those who adopt healthy obsessions about weight control hold themselves to a higher standard. They find it unacceptable to deviate from their plans without dealing with those deviations as problems. This doesn't mean that they berate themselves or abuse themselves when problems develop. It does mean that they see deviations as problems and attempt to deal with them directly. Wouldn't it be great if successful weight control meant having a happy-go-lucky attitude and feeling free of the oppression that seems required for success? It just doesn't work that way. The biology of excess weight is simply too tenacious. It takes a certain level of control, focusing, and intensity to manage it effectively. This leaves little room for happy-go-lucky feelings.

Some of my clients who have lost a lot of weight and kept it off for years have lamented, "Now that I've lost all this weight, I expected to feel good about myself most of the time. But I don't. I still struggle with this every day." Sadly, this is the nature of the battle with the biology of excess weight. Most people do not view their own successes at weight control as joyous accomplishment. People who lose a lot of weight are typically less than trilled about their new weight statuses. Usually, they want to lose another 5, 10, 20, or more pounds. Even if they find their new weights acceptable, they still have to work hard to maintain their focusing. There may be a certain "joy in the discipline." Exercise can bring its own rewards, as can a sense of control about eating patterns. Nevertheless, the state in which many successful weight controllers find themselves feels more like "healthy obsession" than "joyous accomplishment."

## Key Principles

- Almost all of your behaviors are largely controlled by you. Control is not "on" or "off." Control is "more" or "less" in your hands.

- Self-control is the process by which you control your own behaviors in order to achieve desired goals. Self-control involves setting goals and planning, observing, evaluating, rewarding, and punishing your own thoughts and actions.

- Self-control occurs in five phases: (1) problem identification, (2) commitment, (3) execution, (4) environmental management, and (5) generalization.

- Problem identification often involves breaking through denial. Denial is a form of self-protection. Some people who have obvious problems with their weight use denial and convince themselves that change is impossible. Genuine and gentle confrontations, proposals of specific plans for change, and more intensive confrontation with family members can sometimes help these people.

- Methods of improving commitment include using Decision Balance Sheets, using disputing responses, and making commitments public.

- The best outcomes are the result of goals that are defined clearly and specifically; easy when pursuing new or difficult tasks; and moderately challenging or very challenging when pursuing familiar or easy tasks. You must obtain frequent measures of progress toward goals in order to use goals effectively.

- Improving execution of self-control could include establishing long-term plans, using positive self-monitoring, and using mental imagery.

- Moderately specific long-term plans work better than highly specific long-term plans. Making plans for activities on an hourly or daily basis often fail because they are too rigid and don't allow for reasonable fluctuations in daily activities. Weekly or monthly plans produce better results.

- A useful lifetime plan for weight control could include the following steps: (1) try self-directed change; (2) increase involvement of family and friends; (3) join a reasonable weight control program; and (4) join a long-term professional program.

- Positive self-monitoring means systematically gathering information about successes. Negative self-monitoring means systematically gathering information about poor performances. Keeping track of urges that you resist and of exercise sessions may help you maintain effective patterns. After self-monitoring eating and exercise, consider reviewing the most positive aspects of your day's eating and of exercising behaviors. Highlight (by circling or using a colored highlighter) those aspects of the day that were positive or effective.

- You can use imagery for mental rehearsal, preparing for competition, overcoming adversity, managing tension, and increasing commitment. It is best to create images in quiet nondistracting environments and to relax physically before producing images. It also helps to create images that evoke sights, feelings, and emotions as vividly as possible. Imagery works best when it is used very deliberately, with a lot of concentration, and when images are well controlled.

- Effective self-control also involves environmental management. Behavior does not occur in a vacuum. Certain stimuli control or affect patterns of behavior. You can use this principle of stimulus control by decreasing the number of situations in which you allow yourself to eat; placing food only in food areas (kitchen, dining room); discontinuing non-eating activities in food areas; and making eating a "pure experience." Keeping your home safe from problematic foods is another way in which you can manage your environment to promote better self-control.

- In the generalization phase of self-control, weight controllers must transfer the skills they used to lose weight into new situations over long periods of time. Research and experience suggest a variety of ideas, techniques, and issues that affect generalization of self-control: (1) lapse versus relapse; (2) management of injuries and illnesses; (3) scale phobia; (4) permanent vacations; (5) changes in key relationships; (6) work or financial crises; (7) major changes in eating environments; (8) direct versus indirect problem solving; (9) abstinence violation effect (AVE); and (10) healthy obsession. Development of a healthy obsession means feeling extremely committed to a healthy pattern of eating, exercising, and self-monitoring. Persistent weight controllers find disruptions in these patterns quite annoying, and they work hard to resolve the disruptions as quickly as possible.

# Epilogue

B. F. Skinner wrote a powerful and provocative novel about a utopian society created from scientific principles, Walden Two. Skinner's guide to this new world was Frazier. Frazier described the Walden Two approach to helping children develop self-control to an incredulous visitor, Mr. Castle, in several interesting passages (pages 107-109):

"Take the principle of 'Get thee behind me Satan' ... It's a special case of self-control by altering the environment ... We give each child a lollipop which has been dipped in powdered sugar so that a single touch of the tongue can be detected. We tell him he may eat the lollipop later in the day, provided it hasn't already been licked. Since the child is only three or four, it is fairly diff——"

"Three or four!" Castle exclaimed.

"All our ethical training is completed by the age of six," said Frazier quietly.

"A simple principle like putting temptation out of sight would be acquired before four, but at such an early age the problem of not licking the lollipop isn't easy. Now what would you do, Mr. Castle, in a similar situation?"

"Put the lollipop out of sight as quickly as possible."

"Exactly. I see you've been well-trained ... The children are urged to examine their own behavior while looking at the lollipops. This helps them to recognize the need for self-control. Then the lollipops are concealed and the children are asked to notice any gain in happiness or reduction in tension. Then a strong distraction is arranged— say, an interesting game. Later the children are reminded of the candy and encouraged to examine their reaction. The value of the distraction is generally obvious. [The children find they can resist the temptation better when they are distracted] ... When the experiment is repeated a day or so later, the children all run with the lollipops to the lockers and do exactly what Mr. Castle would do—a sufficient indication of the success of our training."

"[In another of our experimental approaches to training self-control] a group of children arrive home after a long walk tired and hungry. They're expecting supper. They find, instead, that it's time for a lesson in self-control: they must stand for five minutes in front of steaming bowls of soup.

"The assignment is accepted like a problem in arithmetic. Any groaning or complaining is a wrong answer. Instead, the children begin at once to work upon themselves to avoid any unhappiness during the delay. One of them may make a joke of it. We encourage a sense of humor as a good way of not taking an annoyance seriously. The joke won't be much, according to adult standards— perhaps the children will simply pretend to empty the bowl of soup into his upturned mouth. Another may start a song with many verses. The rest join in at once, for they have learned that it's a good way to make the time pass.

"[Does this] also strike you as a form of torture? Mr. Castle" Frazier asked.

"I'd rather be put on the rack," said Castle.

"Then you have by no means had the thorough training I supposed. You can't imagine how lightly the children take such an experience. It's a rather severe biological frustration, for the children are tired and hungry and they must stand and look at food; but it's passed off as lightly as a five-minute delay at curtain time. We regard it as a fairly elementary test."

The children in *Walden Two* learned to use distractions during temptations and stimulus control to avoid temptations. These skills remain critically important self-control skills today for persistent weight controllers.

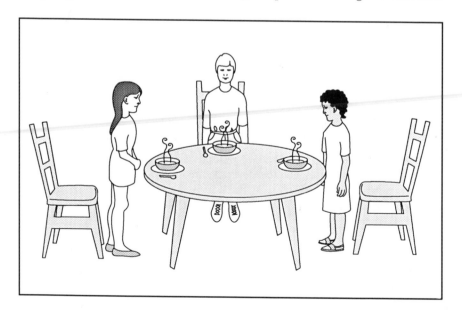

# 8

# Stress and Coping

### The Stressed-Out Weight Control Blues

I've got the stressed-out weight control blues.
Everything is tense,
Feel too many stressors,
Beating on my sense.

Focus has been relentless.
Pushing me past kin,
All those expectations,
Have just done me in.

Calories, fat grams, exercise, exercise,
Monitoring everything in my life.
As demands from bosses and family sit there screeching,
Through me like a knife.

People who used to support me,
Friends once in the past,
Now offer me compliments and cookies,
How long can this last?

Got the stressed-out weight control blues,
So I just sit and stare,
Feel too many stressors,
And no one seems to care.

(Adapted from Whiton
Paine's "The Burnout Blues")

Success usually requires effective management of demands from the environment and from within. Performing well on the job, in school, in sports, and in weight control all share this challenge. Take a minute to think about the successful achievements of your life. You probably managed various aspects of your life effectively while you were succeeding. Friends and family may have supported you. You probably found ways of managing the emotional challenges that you faced at that time. This chapter provides ideas to help you apply those stress management and coping skills to weight control. It begins by defining stress and stressors and describing types of stressors. Then it focuses on how to manage stress and improve coping skills.

## Stress and Stressors

### Definitions

The term "stress" describes complex emotional responses to challenging situations or events. The term "stressor" describes the cause of those reactions. More generally, demands from the environment are considered stressors. Complex emotional responses resulting from experiences with stressors are defined as stress. In most cases, stress includes feelings such as frustration, tension, irritability, hostility, or anger.

### Degrees of Stress

Check the stress responses that you have experienced in the last two weeks from the following list.

---

### Stress Responses

| Physical | Emotional |
|---|---|
| _____ appetite change | _____ anxiety |
| _____ fatigue | _____ frustration |
| _____ sleep problems | _____ anger |
| _____ headaches | _____ mood swings |
| _____ weight change | _____ temper tantrums |
| _____ colds | _____ nightmares |
| _____ stomach upset | _____ crying spells |
| _____ muscle aches | _____ irritability |
| _____ heart pounding | _____ blues |

_____ physical accidents

_____ teeth grinding

_____ restlessness

_____ skin problems

_____ foot-tapping

_____ finger-drumming

_____ increased drug, alcohol, tobacco use

_____ depression

_____ worrying

_____ discouragement

_____ unhappiness

_____ emptiness

_____ cynicism

_____ apathy

**Mental**

_____ unproductive

_____ forgetful

_____ bored

_____ dullness of senses

_____ confusion

_____ poor concentration

_____ nothing matters

_____ silly mistakes

_____ ineffective

**Interpersonal**

_____ distrustful

_____ isolated

_____ intolerant

_____ resentful

_____ lonely

_____ overly critical

_____ clamming up

_____ decreased sex drive

_____ nagging

_____ decreased intimacy

_____ using people

_____ cynical

_____ unforgiving

_____ decreased contacts with friends

If you checked many or most of these items, you are experiencing a high level of stress. These unhappy and frustrated feelings can make the "aggressive self-protectiveness" needed for successful weight control difficult to obtain. How can you make time in your life for exercise, keep your food choices in control, and stay focused and optimistic about weight control in the face of these unhappy feelings and reactions?

The impact of stress increases when stress persists for long periods of time. Repeated exposures to mild stressors or long-lasting exposure to more severe stressors can interfere markedly with your ability to function effectively in any domain (including weight control). Hans Selye conducted research on these reactions. He proposed a model to help describe what happens to your body in response to stressors. Selye called his model the General Adaptation Syndrome, or GAS. The figure shows the three major stages of the GAS and your bodily reactions over time. (This figure is adapted from a figure in *The Stress of Life*, by H. Selye.)

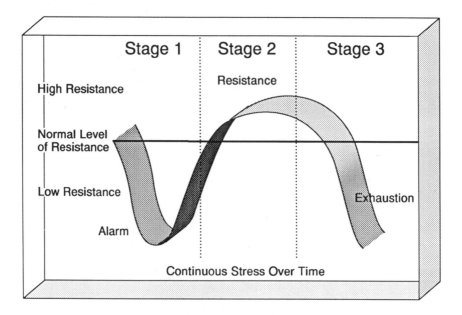

**General Adaptation Syndrome (GAS)**

In the first stage ("alarm and mobilization"), physical resistance to stressors declined rapidly. The nervous system automatically reacts in this stage, placing many demands on your physical resources. For example, the brain, in particular the part of the brain called the hypothalamus, directs the adrenal gland to secrete adrenaline rapidly into the bloodstream. Heart and breathing rates respond by increasing rapidly. This supplies your muscles with more energy (oxygen), allowing you to "fight or flee" as needed. This often results in a state of great tension and alertness and many efforts to cope with the stressor.

Consider your reaction to a major conflict in your family or at work. You may have become obsessed with the problem and focused on it so intensely that you didn't sleep or eat. You may have called your friends about it or talked to yourself about it, ignoring other normal aspects of your life. What happened to your exercise program or your focus on low-fat eating during this extremely stressful time? Most people place weight control on the back burner of their lives during these times. Some weight controllers react during the "alarm and mobilization" stage of the GAS by abandoning their patterns of low-fat, low-sugar eating. Suddenly, brownies, cookies, and burgers become acceptable in a "nothing else matters" reaction to this major stressor. Obviously, this is a dangerous time for weight controllers. Once it becomes acceptable to eat these foods and abandon exercise, the shift in momentum becomes hard to fix.

The body continues to defend against or resist negative effects of stressors in stage two of the GAS ("resistance"). During this stage, powerful hormones, glucocorticoids, are released into the bloodstream. These substances increase the availability of blood sugar to help the body maintain a high level of resistance. Unfortunately, these glucocorticoids also interfere with the body's ability to ward off disease and protect itself against damage in other ways. In other words, your body helps you sustain your ability to adjust to stressors during the "resistance" stage. Unfortunately, as time goes on and you continue battling with these powerful stressors, you begin to lose the ability to resist the negative effects of this struggle (see the "exhaustion stage," stage three in the GAS figure). Studies of prisoners of war and Nazi concentration camp survivors clearly document this GAS pattern. Survivors of such long-lasting and severe stressors often show significant signs of stage three deterioration. What would you feel if you found yourself suddenly out of a job and desperately seeking a way to maintain your household? You might notice stage three reactions over periods of weeks and months. These reactions could include severe anxiety, severe depression, nightmares, impaired sexual potency and interest, and "functional diarrhea" (diarrhea that occurs in response to even brief exposures to mild stressors).

## Types of Stressors

All stressors seem unpredictable and/or uncontrollable. People seem unable to predict when these significant events might befall them. Also, when some stressors occur, people often feel unable to control what they will do. For example, you cannot predict when a police officer will pull you over for a traffic violation. You also cannot control whether or not the police officer will write a ticket or simply give you a warning. In a similar vein, soldiers cannot predict when the enemy will strike and are unable to control events once the fighting starts. In both cases, stress follows events that seem largely unpredictable and uncontrollable.

Think for a moment about events that caused you stress. You may notice that some of them seemed more uncontrollable than unpredictable, or vice versa. Your dog barks whenever a cat strolls by. You cannot predict when a cat will appear, but you can control your dog's barking once it starts. On the other hand, the fact that the 5:00 P.M. traffic produces noise and annoyances is very predictable. But it is impossible for you to control. Because many events are unpredictable, or uncontrollable, or both, it would take hundreds of pages to discuss them all. Instead, let's consider how major "life events" and minor "daily hassles" affect you.

## Major Life Events

The following table is reprinted from "The Social Readjustment Rating Scale," by T. H. Holmes and R. H. Rahe. Think about the past six months of your life. On the table, check the events that you experienced during this period. Add up the numbers under the "Life Change Units" column for each of the events that you checked.

| Major Life Events as Stressors | |
| --- | --- |
| **Life Event** | **Life Change Units** |
| *Family* | |
| Death of spouse | 100 |
| Divorce | 73 |
| Marital separation | 65 |
| Death of close family member | 63 |
| Marriage | 50 |
| Marital reconciliation | 45 |
| Major change in health of family | 44 |
| Pregnancy | 40 |
| Addition of new family member | 39 |
| Major change in arguments with spouse | 35 |
| Son or daughter leaving home | 29 |
| In-law troubles | 29 |
| Spouse starting or ending work | 26 |
| Major change in family get-togethers | 15 |
| *Personal* | |
| Detention in jail | 63 |
| Major personal injury or illness | 53 |
| Sexual difficulties | 39 |
| Death of close friend | 37 |

| | |
|---|---|
| Outstanding persoal achievement | 28 |
| Start or end of formal schooling | 26 |
| Major change in living conditions | 25 |
| Major revision of personal habits | 24 |
| Changing to a new school | 20 |
| Change in residence | 20 |
| Major change in recreation | 19 |
| Major change in church activities | 19 |
| Major change in sleeping habits | 15 |
| Vacation | 13 |
| Christmas | 12 |
| Minor violations of the law | 11 |
| *Work* | |
| Being fired from work | 47 |
| Retirement from work | 45 |
| Major business adjustment | 39 |
| Changing to different line of work | 36 |
| Major change in work responsibilities | 29 |
| Trouble with boss | 23 |
| Major change in working conditions | 20 |
| Total | |

Reasearch suggests that if the total number of your "life change units" was between 0 and 100 you would be expected to get about 1.4 illnesses during the past six months. If you scored over 500, you would have been likely to get twice as many illnesses.

You probably noticed that Holmes and Rahe included several very positive events in their list of life events. Outstanding personal achievements and vacations are two of those positive events. Such positive events certainly could disrupt the normal flow of your life. Recent research shows, however, that people enjoy these positive events and that they usually produce very little stress.

Far more negative life events, such as divorce, deaths in the family, and being fired from work potentially produce much more stress for most people. Nathan Zilberg and his associates conducted a study on the reactions of 72 people to the death of one of their parents. Their research showed that people varied tremendously in their stress responses to such negative life events. The responses of 35 mostly middle-aged people who had sought professional assistance ("patients") are compared in the following table with 37 other people who did not seek professional help to deal with their losses. Six questions are presented here. Note that the patient group reported more stress on each item. Both groups experienced similar major uncontrollable life events. Yet this unfortunate event produced much more impact for one group than the other group.

The people in the study rated each of the following questions on a 4-point scale. From 1 for not at all, to 4 for often. The table gives the average score for each group on each question.

| Questions About Impact | Patients | Nonpatients |
|---|---|---|
| 1. I thought about it when I didn't mean to. | 3.5 | 2.6 |
| 2. I tried not to talk about it. | 2.6 | 0.7 |
| 3. I stayed away from reminders of it. | 2.1 | 1.0 |
| 4. I had waves of strong feelings about it. | 3.8 | 1.9 |
| 5. My feelings about it were kind of numb. | 2.5 | 1.2 |
| 6. Pictures about it popped into my mind. | 3.5 | 2.4 |

Zilberg's research shows that people vary dramatically in the thoughts and feelings they have following traumatic life events. Think about how your friends have reacted when an important personal relationship broke up. One friend may have rehashed what went wrong and felt severely rejected and depressed. Another friend in the same situation may have recovered quickly and tried to find another partner. In a similar vein, some people get very upset and involved when the United States participates in a military action. They become absorbed with the event, watch the news late into the evening, and find it extremely distressing. Other people take such national emergencies much more lightly. Perceptions of the importance of life events and other aspects of personality can dramatically affect the degree to which major life events produce stress.

### Burnout

Some stressful life events take place more gradually than the ones that Holmes and Rahe focused on in their research. Stressors on the job represent a critical example of this type of life event. If you ever saw a house that was burned out, you know what an awful sight it is. What was once a vital structure became empty and deserted. Where there was once activity, happiness, and excitement, only crumbling reminders of energy and life remain. Some parts of the outer structure may still stand. But if you ventured inside, you would be struck by the full force of the desolation.

In many ways, people who burn out on the job become like a house ravished by fire. Under constant stress, their inner resources become consumed (remember the GAS model) as if by fire. There is a great emptiness inside of them, although their outer shells may remain unchanged. People in this situation often become emotionally and physically exhausted. Burned out people want to detach themselves from their jobs, schoolwork, marriages, or any area of their lives that have become stressful. They question whether their efforts were ever worthwhile. They become pessimistic about the future.

Burnout often occurs at the workplace. One factor that affects burnout is an extreme level of commitment and dedication to work. You may believe that is what people expect of you. Or you may be very idealistic about your work. This could include believing that if you work hard enough, you can single-handedly relieve the suffering you encounter in others, create immediate progress, or produce enormous profits. Thus, you take on tasks at work to please others or to reach impossible idealistic standards. You may do this without realizing how much time and energy such efforts take.

Think about your current or most recent job. This should be a position in which you worked long enough to understand what it would be like to work there for several years. On the following page, place a check mark next to each of the items listed that accurately describes your work environment. If your work environment scores three or more checks, it may be "burnout prone." Unfortunately, most work environments "pass" this test. (This list is adapted from a list by J. H. Pfefferling and F. M. Eckel in *Job Stress and Burnout*, by W. S. Paine.)

# Work Environment and Burnout

_____ Expectation that everyone should always help everyone else.

_____ Staff should interact mainly with their peers. without readily crossing the boundaries of the hierarchy.

_____ Constant demands for perfection.

_____ Not eager to allow workers to express their grievances.

_____ Expectation that workers should provide extra efforts even for little or no reward.

_____ No reinforcement for suggestions about improving morale.

_____ Repetitive work activities.

_____ Minimal additional help provided for tasks that require extra effort.

_____ Lack of encouragement for showing concern about your mental health.

_____ Discouragement of full participation.

_____ Preachy leadership styles.

_____ Changes in policies emerge without considering the priority of the problem that is being remedied.

_____ Changes in policies occur so frequently there is no time to evaluate them.

_____ Rigid role definitions for workers.

_____ Playfulness is considered unprofessional and inappropriate.

_____ Frequent discrimination against people based on age, sex, race, and relationship to employer.

_____ Emphasis on past successes.

_____ Very little emphasis on positive feedback.

_____ Very little concern about the comfort of the environment.

_____ Enforcement of policies and bases of policies constantly shifting.

### Daily Hassles

Research indicates that daily annoyances or hassles can produce as much stress as more major life events. Consider the degree to which the following hassles affect your feeling of well-being and mood:

- Being interrupted while talking
- Experiencing problems with children
- Being ignored by others
- Having someone break a promise or appointment
- Having minor arguments with spouse, friend, co-worker
- Being embarrassed
- Performing poorly at a task
- Doing something you are unskilled at
- Being unable to complete a task
- Being late
- Failing to understand something
- Having someone fail to knock at your door
- Worrying about someone else's problems
- Being interrupted during a task

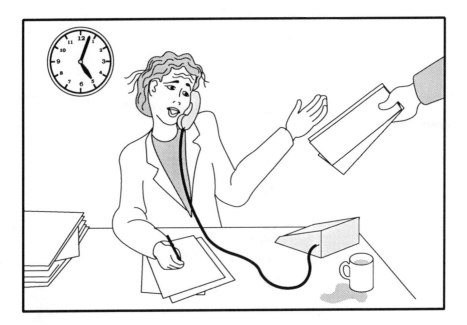

- Being crowded or pushed
- Having a minor accident (broke something, tore clothing)
- Experiencing bad weather
- Having difficulty in traffic
- Being criticized
- Becoming fearful
- Misplacing something
- Forgetting something
- Doing something that you did not want to do

What is your reaction to reading over this list? Perhaps you felt some discomfort just reading and remembering when these events happened to you. People report such unpleasant reactions. When two or more of these events occur in one day, most people react quite negatively. Clearly, both minor daily hassles and major life events produce challenges to your ability to cope and stay focused on weight control.

# Managing Stress

- Why do some people burn out, whereas others thrive in high-stress jobs?
- Why do some people you know become "unglued" by very minor daily hassles, whereas others let almost everything "roll off their backs"?
- Why do major life events devastate some people, whereas the same events seem like minor inconveniences for others?

These questions raise issues about how and why some people manage stress and cope better than others. To understand such differences and help you refine your stress management and coping skills, information about personality characteristics, social support, and stress management and coping skills are considered here.

## Personality Characteristics

Take a moment and think of people you know who always seem to feel under pressure. Now think of individuals who are usually calm and relaxed. How do the personalities of these two groups of people differ? Also, think of people you know who cope very well with personal crises. How are they different from individuals who "fall apart" when the going gets tough? Researchers have asked similar questions and they have identified some remarkable differences among people.

### Type A or Type B

To decide whether you are a Type A or a Type B person, answer the following questions either "yes" or "no":

---

## Type A or Type B

_____ Time passes too quickly for me to accomplish all the things I want to do.

_____ I feel I am under great pressure to achieve.

_____ I become very anxious about completing tasks that are left unfinished.

_____ I have a very high energy level.

_____ I often feel quite hostile toward other people.

_____ I am a very competitive individual.

---

If you answered "yes" to all of these questions, you may well have Type A characteristics. Type A people are hard-driving, energetic, and competitive. They also can become quite hostile or angry when challenged. People with Type B personality characteristics are much more calm, relaxed, and less in a rush to accomplish things.

Ray Rosenman and his co-workers compared Type A with Type B behavior patterns. They showed that Type A people have a higher rate of heart problems. More specifically, they followed a group of 3154 healthy middle-aged men for 8 1/2 years. Type A men were twice as likely as Type B men to develop coronary heart disease.

You may have some Type A characteristics. This certainly does not mean that you will soon experience a heart attack. Actually, more than 50 percent of the population can be classified as Type A. Most of these people will not develop abnormal problems with their hearts. Type A individuals are just somewhat more likely than their less driven, less pressured Type B peers to develop these difficulties.

The root of the problem concerns how you respond to stressors. Type A people respond more rapidly to a greater number of stressors than do Type B people. Their responses also commonly include anger. This means that Type A people experience a greater variety of unpleasant stimuli as stressors. They also react more quickly to everyday stressors than do Type B people. While some people become sad or depressed when reacting to stressors, Type A people often become angry. Many people, for example, react to the death of a loved one with great sadness. Type A people may react with anger about the injustice of death. Unfortunately, both excessive reactions to stressors and more angry reactions are associated with increased heart problems.

These findings indicate that Type A people would benefit from learning more effective ways to manage stress. This could decrease their risk of heart attack. Individuals with Type A characteristics might benefit from getting more support from others and by refining specific skills for coping with stressors. More information about such skills is presented later in this chapter. Another approach that may help Type A people is to develop "hardy" personality characteristics.

### Hardiness

Explorers, pioneers, and lumberjacks seem hardy. But can you imagine a hardy lawyer or a hardy business executive? Suzanne Kobasa and colleagues found quite a few hardy lawyers and business executives. These hardy professionals often did not look like gruff explorers and pioneers, but all of them resembled each other in the way they responded to stressors. Hardy people survive and become more competent under stress.

Three Cs define hardiness: commitment, control, and challenge. To explain these three Cs, consider the case of a male executive who just learned that he had to transfer to a new job in a completely new city. The executive, Mr. Mobile, must now face the challenge of working with new people, finding a new home, helping his family adjust to a new neighborhood and new schools, learning new job skills, and just getting around in a new city. Because Mr. Mobile is *committed*, he approaches this difficult life event with a sense of purpose. He does not passively allow the newness of his surroundings to overwhelm him. Instead, he actively explores the new job and the new city. He and Mrs. Mobile, his wife, spend several hours reading a city map and driving around town to become more familiar with the city. Mr. Mobile even takes the same approach to his new office building. He walks around the building meeting as many new people as possible. Mr. Mobile also sees the new job as another chance for self-improvement. He uses it to learn new skills and to become a better executive. In other words, he finds a purpose or a meaning in the challenge of the new position.

Mr. Mobile sees himself as *controlling* his life. Although the new job places him in a strange new world, he tries to influence what goes on there. He works hard and accomplishes a lot. Mr. Mobile does not believe that he controls everything about this new job but he does know that hard work, listening to other people, and being open to new learning pays off. Mr. Mobile recognizes that he can control at least some important aspects of his environment, regardless of the stressors he encounters.

Mr. Mobile also enjoys the *challenge* of the job transfer. He recognizes that change is normal in life. He views changes as opportunities that challenge him to grow. Some people fear change because they are afraid that they may not be able to function in new and different circumstances. They would rather adjust to stressors than to look for new ways to become competent. Mr. Mobile, on the other hand, seeks competence. Merely "adjusting" bores him.

Kobasa and her associates found that people like Mr. Mobile, who are committed to their lives and work, who believe they can control their fates, and who seek stressors as challenges to their ability to grow, manage stress very effectively. "Hardy" lawyers and executives remain much healthier than their less hardy colleagues even when they are faced with many stressors.

One of my weight control clients demonstrated a less hardy approach to a major conflict at work. This weight controller had been exercising effectively and eating approximately 1200 calories using a low-fat/low-eating plan. When the conflict emerged and became especially severe, she found herself eating a lunch consisting of garlic bread, pasta with heavy cheese sauce, and high-fat ice cream for dessert. She recognized her response to the stressor from work. She continued her self-monitoring, including writing down both calories and fat grams from her problematic lunch. She and I discussed a method of handling the problem at work that she became energized about. She had felt unable to control the conflict at work and felt very victimized by it. After she and I talked, she had an alternative plan that could begin resolving the problem. She felt much better after developing this plan and, for the first time in a week, went for an exercise walk and began sleeping restfully again. The work problem was eventually resolved, as most of these rather severe stressors usually are after a while. My client felt a lot better because she accepted the challenge posed by her problem by taking control of it.

Can you become a hardier person? How can you take charge of your life? How can you attack problems rather than retreat from facing them? Try responding to stressors by asking yourself a few questions that direct you to take charge of the situation. For example, you can ask: "What can I do to eliminate this stressor?" "How can I look at this problem as a potential for growth?" "In what way does this stressor tell me something about my goals in life?" "How can I use this situation to improve my competence?"

Becoming hardier also involves a little help from your friends. Mr. Mobile was not alone when he made the switch from his old job to his new one. His family cared about him. As discussed in the next section, family and friends can help a great deal—especially in the face of stressors.

## Social Support

People need people. This is more than just the subject of a popular song. Research shows that people who have good relationships with others suffer fewer medical and emotional problems than more isolated people. People with good social support even live longer than those without good connections to other people. A study of 7000 adults in Alameda County, California, showed that people who lacked relationships with others died at a younger age than those who were married, had frequent contacts with friends and neighbors, and belonged to social clubs or religious groups. According to various studies, support from others can reduce the effects of several other types of stressors:

- Women who had another person with them during labor and childbirth experienced fewer complications than women who did not have a husband, relative, or friend present. The supported group gave birth sooner, were awake more after delivery, and played with their babies more than the unsupported group.

- Social support helped men who lost their jobs. Men with good support reported fewer illnesses and less depression than men who did not have adequate support from others following the loss of their jobs.

- Support by parents and hospital staff helped children adjust more effectively to the after-effects of surgery.

- The adjustment of people to heart attacks, tuberculosis, and asthma was improved when people had spouses, friends, and relatives around them.

How do your family and friends support you? How do they help? What do they give you or do for you? The way most people answer these questions indicates that they need more than just the presence of other people; they need people around who actively show that they care. People provide social support in three ways. Family and friends provide us with emotional comforting, helpful information, and material goods such as money or food. All three of these qualities of support can help you manage stress effectively.

**Emotional support** People provide me with emotional support when they:

- Listen and talk things over when I want to feel that someone understands me

- Allow me to talk freely about my problems and private thoughts

- Show confidence in me and encourage me

**Informational support** People provide me with informational support when they:

- Give me advice I can count on

- Give me names of people who can do very competent work (good doctors and lawyers, for example)

- Give me good ideas about personal and family problems

**Material support**  People provide me with material support when they:

- Look after my belongings (like my plants or pets) if I have to leave town for a few days

- Help me get to a doctor if I can't get myself to one

- Loan me money when I really need it

Thus, part of stress management includes knowing when and who to ask for help. The next table, on the following page, is adapted from one by N. L. Tubesing and D. H. Tubesing. Fill it in to help clarify who you can and do use for support. When life's little stressors increase, leaning on others helps. Friends and family can provide information, material goods, or emotional support. Their job of helping often becomes easier if you ask for the specific kind of help you want.

Sources of support require some maintenance from you. It is very important to give as well as receive support. To do this, you may wish to look for signs from others that they want your help. Perhaps you already notice when those around you appear stressed. Your "significant others" would probably welcome and appreciate your offers of support under such conditions.

# Coping Skills

Consider your reaction to going to a dentist. Just imagine yourself in your dentist's waiting room:

> There you are sitting in your dentist's waiting room. You nervously look around the room and find other faces nervously looking around the room. You pick up a magazine that is several months old. You have already read this magazine, but you thumb through it anyway. It's something familiar and safe. You try telling yourself to relax. You uneasily notice that toothpastey, mouthwashy, odor. Then you hear the painful, screeching, whining, metallic sound of the drill.

What was your reaction to that image? Many people cringe at the thought of such things. Yet, although stressful, dental and medical treatments keep us healthy. Other situations that do not produce physical pain also produce stress. The idea of making a speech in public, taking a test,

## Personal Supporters

| People Who: | At Home | At Work | At Play |
|---|---|---|---|
| Excite me | | | |
| Calm me | | | |
| Free me | | | |
| Bring me joy | | | |
| Support/nurture me | | | |
| Stimulate/challenge me | | | |
| Give me meaning | | | |
| Make me laugh | | | |
| Energize me | | | |

and many other things may also seem quite painful. Fortunately, there are ways of thinking and behaving in response to stressors that reduce or prevent their unpleasant effects. Called stress management and coping skills, they include:

- The stress inoculation procedure
- The reattribution technique
- Rational emotive therapy techniques
- Assertiveness
- Effective problem solving
- Management of sleep problems

## Stress Inoculation

Donald Meichenbaum developed a useful approach to handling major stressors. He considers stress inoculation as a method that builds "psychological antibodies." Stress inoculation has helped people control anger, improve test-taking, improve interpersonal skills, decrease anxiety from public speaking, decrease anxiety associated with performing music, decrease fear of flying, and improve adaptation to surgery by children and adults. The procedure includes an educational phase, a coping self-talk phase, a relaxation component, and a practice component.

### Education About the Stressor

In this phase, important information about the stressor is provided. For example, children going to their first dental appointment may not know what happens there. A friend may have told them that it hurts or that a big person in a white coat will yank out their teeth with a pair of pliers. Just learning what happens in a real dental visit often helps young patients adapt to that difficult situation. In a similar way, many people lack information about a variety of stressors. Students often do not know the best strategies for taking tests; medical patients often have serious misconceptions about their illnesses or about hospitals and treatments; and, more generally, people often do not ask enough questions to learn about new jobs, new cities, new cars, and other potentially stressful events.

When facing a stressor, ask questions of people who do understand it; read about it; and take other actions to educate yourself about its nature and effects.

### Coping Self-Statements

All people talk to themselves sometimes. Many people think that talking to yourself is a sign of craziness. Actually, the opposite may be more accurate; not talking to yourself may be a sign of craziness. You may have noticed that you "talk yourself into" doing difficult things. Imagine taking your first dive off of a diving board or making your first public speech. You may recall making self-statements like, "C'mon, you can do it." "You know what to do." "Go for it." These statements provide instructions and encouragements that help when facing challenges of all kinds.

Psychologists advise people facing such challenges to use four types of self-statements: preparing for the stressor, confronting and handling the stressor, coping with feelings at critical moments, and rewarding yourself for successful coping. The following lists provide a sampling of these four types of self-statements that you can use to manage almost any stressor. As you can see by the lists, people who use these self-statements actively cope with stressors. This approach encourages you to become a "hardy" coper in the same way that Suzanne Kobasa's hardy lawyers and executives managed stress. Both approaches to stress management encourage you to see stressors as opportunities to exert control and to enjoy and benefit from a challenge.

Think of a stressor that you have faced recently. It could be taking an exam, going to a doctor or dentist, asking for a favor, or performing before an audience. Try to imagine how you would talk yourself into and through these challenges. Then review the following lists of self-statements and see if you could have used some of them to help you manage that stressor.

**Preparing for a stressor**   Thoughts to use before the stressor occurs:

- What do I have to do?
- I can create a plan to deal with this.
- Thinking about what I have to do is certainly better than getting nervous.
- Worrying won't help. Plan.
- My anxiety tells me that I have a challenge facing me.
- I can learn from this.
- Just keep being logical and calm

**Confronting and handling the stressor**   Thoughts to use during the stressor:

- I can handle this.
- I can meet this challenge.
- Just take it one step at a time; follow the plan.
- Beat the fear: Think of what I am doing.
- Relax. I'm in control. Just take a slow deep breath. Ah . . .
- My tension just tells me to follow my plan; deal with this challenge.

**Coping with feelings at critical moments** Thoughts to help control excess tension during the stressor:

- When tension comes, just pause and breathe slowly.
- Focus on the present. Now what do I have to do?
- I've handled this before and can manage it now.
- I'll rate my fear from one to ten and then watch it change.
- I'll just keep the tension manageable; I won't worry about eliminating it altogether.
- I can do this. It will be over in a certain amount of time.
- Okay, keep focused on what I want to do.
- This is the worst thing that can happen.
- Remember, I don't have to handle this perfectly, just reasonably well.
- Focus on the sensations here: coldness, warmth, smells, touch, taste, sights, and sounds.
- Think about other times and places. Good feelings come with good thoughts.
- I'm in control.

**Rewarding yourself for successful coping** Congratulate yourself for successful management of a difficult situation—after it's over:

- Nice going? I was able to do it.
- It wasn't as tough as I expected.
- Wait till I tell (a friend, spouse, other family member) about it.
- I'm making progress.
- My plan worked.
- I'm learning all the time.
- It's my thinking that creates tension. When I control my self-statements, I can control my tension.
- I'm doing better each time I use these self-statements.
- I'm really pleased with my progress.

### Learning To Relax

Some of the coping self-statements provide reminders about how to relax when dealing with stressors. Learning to relax could involve taking slow, deep breaths, meditating, taking a catnap, tensing and relaxing specific muscles, taking a hot bath, stretching, and getting regular exercise and adequate sleep.

John Stevens described a particularly good method of learning to relax that you could use to reduce or prevent stress. Try the following breathing exercise and see if you feel more calm and relaxed after doing it:

> Focus your attention on your breathing. . . . Become aware
> of all the details or your breathing. . . . Feel the air moving
> into your lungs through either your nose or mouth. . . .
> Notice how your chest and stomach expand and contract
> gently as you breathe. . . . Tune in to your body as you
> breathe. . . . Now imagine that instead of you breathing air,
> that air is breathing you. Imagine the air gently moving
> into your lungs . . . ; then slowly withdrawing. . . . You don't
> have to do anything at all, because the air is breathing for
> you. . . . Just experience the air breathing you for a while.

For another "breathing exercise," just take a slow, deep breath and then slowly exhale. Inhale and say, "One," paying attention to your lungs filling with air. Exhale and say "One."

Edmund Jacobson developed a more elaborate technique called "progressive muscle relaxation." It consists of a series of exercises that involve tensing muscle groups and then relaxing them. By first tensing a muscle, it is much easier to "let it go" and relax it. With your muscles becoming more and more relaxed, it is easier for you to calm down and be in control of your behavior.

> Sit in a comfortable chair in a quiet room with low light.
> Close your eyes and then focus your attention on various
> muscle groups— alternating with tension and relaxation.
> Settle back in the chair, take a deep breath, let it out slowly,
> close your eyes, and make your mind a complete blank.
> Extend your arms directly in front of you, clench your fists
> and tighten all the muscles in your arms. Tense your
> muscles about 3/4 of the maximum that you could tighten
> them. This is enough to feel quite a bit of tension without
> risking injury. Hold this for 5 seconds, then say "Relax," as
> you let your arms slide to the arms of the chair and relax.
> Focus on the immediate contrast between the tension that
> was in your arms and the developing relaxation. Let your
> arms and hands relax for 30 to 60 seconds. During this
> time, you might notice the relaxation developing and how
> your hands and arms feel different from the rest of your
> body. Repeat this procedure for a second time, tensing for 5
> seconds and relaxing for 30 to 60 seconds.

Follow the same procedure for other muscle groups (remembering to use 3/4 tension in all cases) as described next.

- **Face.** Squint your eyes, crease your forehead, and clench your teeth. Hold the tension for 5 seconds, then "Relax." Notice the relaxation develop over your face. Keep relaxing for 30 to 60 seconds. Repeat the procedure.

- **Upper trunk.** Take a deep breath, shrug your shoulders, and tense the muscles in your chest, neck, and back. Hold the tension for 5 seconds, then "Relax." Notice the relaxation develop over your upper trunk. Keep relaxing for 30 to 60 seconds. Repeat the procedure.

- **Lower trunk and legs.** Lift your legs five inches off the floor and tighten your stomach and buttocks and all the muscles in your legs. Hold the tension for 5 seconds, then "Relax." Notice the relaxation develop over your lower trunk and legs. Keep relaxing for 30 to 60 seconds. Repeat the procedure.

After you have practiced this routine several times in a relaxed environment, you will notice that it becomes easier and easier to become totally relaxed in shorter and shorter periods of time. When you are able to relax yourself in a reasonably short period of time (three minutes or less) you are ready to begin using relaxation as a tool to combat periods of tension and stress. When you notice the tension and stress building, consider it a signal for you to focus on the feelings of tension in your body. Quickly tense your muscles, release, and then relax.

Nancy and Donald Tubesing developed the "ten-second break" technique that appears on the following page. Many people find it very useful.

You can also use your imagination to take yourself away to a beach or summer cottage. All of these devices can help prevent little hassles from becoming big stressors.

### Practicing

Managing stress requires practice in the same way that a sport, driving, typing, or mastering any new skill does. Many people don't deliberately talk to themselves—especially when facing stressors. Practicing what to say to yourself at critical moments can help you cope with surgery, manage pain, or become a more skillful athlete. In all of these applications, practicing the use of coping self-statements helps people adapt to stress. Practicing relaxation also helps reduce stress. You will find that practicing breathing exercises, meditation, yoga, or any other method helps make relaxation more natural and comfortable.

Karl Kirkland and James Hollandsworth showed that the effective use of stress management skills can improve performance on exams. Answer the questions in the Managing Stress questionnaire about taking an

## Ten-Second Relaxation Break

**Basic Routine**

Step 1 — Smile as you think to yourself "My body doesn't need this _____.
(irritation or stress)

Step 2 — Take a slow, deep belly breath—
Count to 4 slowly on the inhale and on the exhale.

Step 3 — Take a second deep belly breath—
Close your eyes at the top of the inhalation.
As you exhale . . . imagine (visualize or feel) something warm entering your body at your head . . . and flow down into your hands and feet. Heaviness and warmth are flowing in. Think the phrase, "I am calm."

Step 4 — Open your eyes.

**Modified Routine for Phone Calls**

Step A — When the phone begins to ring.
Do Step 3 (above) first—then answer the phone.

Step B — During the phone call:
Relax your shoulders and jaw.
Breathe from your abdomen as rhythmically as possible.

Step C — After the phone call:
Do the complete ten-second break, Steps 1 through 4.

exam using the information that's been presented on stress management skills. Then check your answers against the ones provided to see how well you used the information.

### Suggested Stress Management Skills for Taking a Test

**Education.** Budgeting time is an important aspect of dealing with exams effectively. First discover how much time is allotted for the entire exam and then calculate how much time is allotted for each section of

# Managing Stress

**Stressor: Taking a test**

Education:
What are the important facts that apply to taking any exam?
Answer:

Coping self-statements:
Preparing for the stressor: How can I prepare for an exam?
Answer:

Confronting and handling the stressor:
What should I do to manage the stress I feel as I begin an exam?
Answer:

Coping with feelings at critical moments:
How do I avoid panicking?
Answer:

Rewarding yourself for successful coping:
How should I react after successfully finishing the exam?
Answer:

Relaxation:
How can I improve my ability to relax and generally take care of myself?
Answer:

Practice:
When and how should I practice these stress management skills for taking an exam?
Answer:

the exam, or decide about how many questions you should answer in the first quarter of the exam, and so on. Watching for key words and understanding them is another important aspect of tests. Phrases like "compare and contrast," "all of the following," and "define" tell you some important things about the question. Every college and university counseling center and library have many books in test taking. Why not read more about it?

**Coping self-statements preparing for the stressor.** Develop a workable plan for studying. consider what you have to accomplish in the time between now and the exam. Make a schedule that shows what you will do for this exam and for your other courses for each week before the exam.

**Confronting and handling the stressor.** Talk to yourself in a calm manner and direct your attention to the task at hand. You can tell yourself to relax, take a slow deep breath, and realize that you have already prepared for this test. Now all you have to do is answer the questions as well as possible. Think of it as a challenge or a puzzle. (Remember how "hardy" lawyers would handle this.) Focus on the steps needed to complete the exam. First, put your name on the answer sheets. Then plan your time for each section of the exam. Finally, begin answering the questions. Answer only those you believe you know at first. Skip the ones you feel unsure of. You can come back to those at the end of the exam.

**Coping with feelings at critical moments.** When you feel very tense or panicky, use that feeling as a reminder to talk to yourself according to your plan. You may feel very tense. You may think, "I will flunk. I will be kicked out of school. My parents will be ashamed of me. What will I do with my life?" These thoughts do not help you manage the task at hand. If you are feeling panicky and thinking about such things, remind yourself what to say to yourself. Focus your attention back onto the pieces of paper in front of you. Try taking a deep breath and relaxing. Tell yourself you can only take your best shot here and how. The future will have to wait until after the exam.

**Rewarding things to say.** You made it! Even if you did not get the highest grade possible, you got through it without falling apart. You finished it and followed your plan. You can be proud of that accomplishment.

**Relaxation.** First, be sure to stay with your eating plan and get plenty of rest. Second, use meditation, breathing techniques, or other relaxation procedures.

**Practice.** As soon a you know when an exam is scheduled, you can begin to develop a plan to prepare for it. Several weeks before the exam, try reviewing all of these skills one or two times per week. Practice your relaxation techniques and use them when you feel especially tense before or during the exam.

Some situations require more stress inoculation than others for most weight controllers. Coping with these high-risk situations successfully can maintain momentum and prevent serious lapses. To help you identify which situations pose problems for you, read the list of high-risk situations in the following table. Can you think of other ways in which you struggle to cope? Next, to help you think of ways to cope with these situations, look at the list of coping responses that follows the table. For each situation in the table that creates problems for you, list all of the coping response item numbers that might help you handle the problem. Can you think of other ways to cope with your high-risk situations?

Now read through the following coping responses and fill in the numbers that might help you handle the high-risk situations in the table.

## Handling High-Risk Situations

| High-Risk Situations | Coping Responses |
|---|---|
| Getting home from work | _____ |
| During the weekend | _____ |
| Watching TV | _____ |
| Studying or reading | _____ |
| Eating at your family's home (for example, at your parents' home) | _____ |
| During the holidays (especially Halloween, Thanksgiving, Christmas, Hanukkah) | _____ |
| Being around someone who is encouraging you to eat something high in fat and sugar that you like. | _____ |
| Wanting to eat something when only high-calorie foods are available | _____ |
| Seeing/smelling problematic foods you like | _____ |
| Being at a party or social gathering | _____ |
| Eating in restaurants | _____ |
| Attending business functions where food and drink are available | _____ |
| During coffee break | _____ |
| When someone brings high-fat food into the office (cookies, muffins, pizza) | _____ |
| Lunches at work | _____ |

| High-Risk Situations | Coping Responses |
|---|---|
| Being alone and/or feeling lonely | _____ |
| When you feel blue, down, and depressed | _____ |
| When you feel frustrated and angry | _____ |
| When you are bored | _____ |
| When you feel stressed and pressured | _____ |
| When you are happy and relaxed | _____ |
| After you have stuck to your weight control plan for several days and feel like rewarding yourself for your hard work | _____ |
| After you have lost several pounds and feel you deserve to take it easy | _____ |
| After you have not stuck to your weight control plan and think you have blown the program | _____ |
| When you are hungry | _____ |
| When you crave something | _____ |
| _____ | _____ |
| _____ | _____ |
| _____ | _____ |

1. Leave the situation.

2. Call or talk to someone (for example, a friend, brother, sister).

3. Think about the reasons you want to control your weight and the benefits that will result from being thinner.

4. Exercise.

5. Do something enjoyable to distract yourself (for example, read a good book or magazine, visit a friend, listen to music, do a crossword puzzle, see a movie).

6. Make your lunch and bring it with you.

7. Eat some low-calorie snacks that will fill you up (for example, carrots, celery, plain popcorn).

8. Drink a lot of water or other very low-calorie fluids (for example, noncaffeinated drinks such as diet soda, club soda with lemon or lime, bouillon, and herbal teas).

9. Write an entry in a journal, diary, or letter that allows you to ventilate your feelings.

10. Reward yourself in ways other than eating food (for example, buy something inexpensive such as a tape, record, or book; go somewhere pleasant like a movie, a friend's home, a park, or a sporting event; or do something else you enjoy like walking, dancing, or a favorite hobby).

11. Keep your home supplied with foods appropriate for your weight control effort and eliminate foods you are trying to avoid or limit.

12. Shop for groceries on the weekend and cook meals for the week.

13. Keep a food diary.

14. Wait a half-hour until the hunger or craving passes.

15. Forgive yourself. Controlling weight is very hard to do. When a slip or lapse happens, apply the brakes quickly and get back on track. A minor slip does not have to become a major disaster.

16. Remind yourself of all the negative consequences of being overweight.

17. Order lower-fat, lower-calorie foods.

18. Bring something you can eat with you (for example, low-calorie snacks for work, raw vegetable plate with a "lite" dip to a party).

19. Do something to relax (for example, think of something pleasurable; take a shower or bath; make a plan about how you will approach the problem).

20. Suggest going to a place where appropriate food choices exist.

21. Tell yourself, "Stop!" before you get swept away by the situation. Focusing on the situation and your goal immediately will improve your ability to deal with it successfully.

22. Meet your family or friends after they are out of the situation you find hard to handle.

23. Talk to your therapist and group members about the high-risk situation and have them help you come up with ways to cope with it.

24. Focus on an image of yourself as a thinner and healthier person who can control his or her eating very effectively.

25. Become involved in after-work or weekend activities (for example, going to a concert or museum, doing volunteer work).

26. Eat a low-calorie snack before going to a social or business function or restaurant.

27. Chew sugar-free gum.

28. Spray breath freshener in your mouth or brush your teeth.

29. Use something during the week to remind yourself of your weight control effort (for example, a colored dot placed on your watch; carry a picture of yourself as a thinner, healthier person).

30. Remind yourself that all food counts. Giving yourself permission because "I've blown it already today" just makes weight control more difficult.

31. _____
    _____

32. _____
    _____

## Reattribution Technique

Attributions are beliefs about the causes of behavior. These beliefs attribute responsibility for actions or thoughts. The reattribution technique involves changing your attributions about problems or lapses into hopeful ways of thinking about them.

Attributions vary along three dimensions:

**Internal-External**
**Stable-Unstable**
**Global-Specific**

*Internal attributions* ascribe causes of events to yourself. *External attributions* ascribe the primary cause for events or behaviors on others or the environment. For example, what if someone who was trying to change her eating and exercising habits ate several handfuls of peanuts and two desserts at a party. She could blame herself exclusively for the problem ("I am just very weak and I don't want to change.") Or she could decide that the party was a "high-risk situation" that she did not manage effectively. Viewing the party as a problematic situation places some of the blame for the difficulty she encountered on the environment, thereby making an external attribution.

*Stable attributions* are those that assert that causes remain relatively consistent over time. If you gained weight last week, you could decide that you just don't have the willpower to lose weight. Or you could believe that you do not really care about losing weight. More useful, *unstable attributions* for the weight gain imply that changes will occur over time, such as: "I had a particularly stressful week; I could have focused on planning and exercising more thoroughly than I did last week."

*Global attributions* assign responsibilities for behaviors and events in very general terms. For example, imagine that you just worked hard at weight control all week and then did not lose any weight. You could decide that your weight stayed the same because "life isn't fair" or "that is just the way it goes sometimes." These are very general beliefs about the causes of your problem. More specific attributions include "the scale is an imperfect measure of change"; or "perhaps I did not exercise as much as I thought I did"; or "perhaps I ate more than I thought I did."

The most helpful attributions are those that keep you hopeful. Therefore, when you are making good progress toward changes in eating and exercising (and weight loss), try to attribute that progress to yourself (internal attribution). It also helps to avoid making internal, global, and stable attributions for problems or lapses. If you believe that something within you causes you problems that you cannot change, you will certainly increase your chances of failure. When you encounter problems, or "failures," try to find the *external* factors that contributed to them. Work toward realizing that the causes of the problem are *specific* factors that can change. Remember, this reattribution technique does not simply rationalize or blindly explain away problems. It helps you stay hopeful by encouraging you to view lapses in perspective.

## Rational Emotive Therapy (RET) Techniques

Here are some common irrational beliefs:

- A person should be loved, or approved of, by almost everyone.

- In order to be worthwhile, a person should be competent in almost all respects.

- Things should always be exactly the way I want them to be; it's terrible when they're not.

- A person should be (that is, needs to be) dependent upon other stronger individuals.

- A person's present and future behavior is irreversibly dependent on significant events from the past.

- Every problem has (should have; must have) an ideal solution; it is catastrophic when the solution is not found.

If you believe these statements and live by them, you will undoubtedly become anxious or depressed quite often. Albert Ellis developed the idea that accepting irrational beliefs as ultimate truths can create unpleasant emotions. You can recognize the irrational beliefs by the language used when stating them. In the examples above, several statements include the word "should" and "needs to" and "must have." Albert Ellis suggested that these terms limit choices. These terms are "absolute-isms" or "categorical imperatives." When you tell yourself you "have to," "should," and "ought to" do something, you tell yourself that you have very few choices. The more rules you force yourself to follow, the less freedom you experience. Almost everyone rebels against restrictions in their freedom. The experience of restricted freedom is highly stressful.

Other words that suggest irrational thinking include all, always, awful, essential, every, horrible, terrible, and totally. These words *exaggerate* problems or concerns. Such exaggerations contribute to a feeling of helplessness. You may recall an earlier discussion emphasizing the importance of active problem solving for maintaining weight change. Using language and beliefs that encourage helplessness leads to giving up.

When you recognize yourself using absolute-isms or exaggerations, you can reactivate your problem solving by disputing these irrational beliefs. Consider the following examples of irrational beliefs and the disputing responses that can modify them appropriately.

| Irrational Beliefs | Disputing Responses (Counterarguments) |
|---|---|
| I'll never be able to lose all of this weight. | I've got to begin somewhere. I can start by focusing on the first five pounds. If I don't try, I'll probably continue to gain weight and feel worse about it. |
| I look awful. I can never lose enough weight to look decent. | It doesn't help to "awfulize." Certainly people don't stop in the street and faint because of my looks. I look okay. I'm just overweight and that creates problems for me. Other people have been successful in losing weight, so why can't I? If I take it one step at a time, I can get there. |
| I've lost eight pounds and no one even noticed. | Probably someone has noticed, even if they haven't said something to me. Commenting on someone's weight loss can be rude. Some people say things like, "you look so much better!" That implies that you looked lousy before losing the weight. I've noticed the weight loss and can feel it in my clothes and my energy level. That's as important as anything. |
| I have to lose weight fast. | Of course, I'd prefer to lose weight quickly. Who wouldn't? If I lose weight slowly and steadily, I'll get to where I want to be. I haven't exercised much for the last several years, and my eating has included too much fat and too much sugar. It took a long time for this pattern to develop and it will take a while to change it. |

| | |
|---|---|
| I'll gain back all the weight I've lost and then some. | Managing weight is very challenging. I'm still learning to manage my weight, and lapses from time to time are typical. I can expect some fluctuations in weight. That doesn't mean I will ultimately be unsuccessful. It makes very little sense to predict failure when the future is not known to anyone. |
| I'm afraid others will see me as a failure. | Not everyone is concerned about my weight. Many people can respect how hard I try. Being overly concerned with others' opinions of me is a burden I don't want. I can choose to ignore what others say and appreciate what I accomplish. |
| I'm afraid I won't like myself after I've lost the weight. | Making arbitrary, negative predictions about the future won't benefit me. I am much more than my weight. There are many things I like about myself. I can feel good about my success and my improved health by staying on track. |
| I can't stand it when people compliment me. | I really *can* stand it. I don't enjoy it. Some people who offer compliments recognize the hard work required to lose weight. I don't have to think of their remarks as a pressure or burden. I can decide to what extent I will pressure myself to manage my weight. |
| It's absolutely impossible for me to resist these (cookies). I really love them. | How can I love a cookie? A cookie is butter and sugar and flavorings. It's not a person and "loving it" just gets in my way. It is certainly possible for me to resist these cookies. If someone offered me a million dollars to give up these cookies for the rest of my life, I wouldn't eat these cookies. I can do it for myself as well as for some make-believe reward. I have the power to resist eating anything I want to. |
| I can't stand being a fanatic every day of my life. | First of all, I can stand it. Second of all, no one says I must do everything every single day. I can back off some days and be more aggressive on others. |

| | |
|---|---|
| I shouldn't be concerned about what others think of me. | Humans are social creatures. It's reasonable for me to be concerned about the opinions of others. It's unreasonable for me to think that I must live my life based on the opinions of others. I can make choices about how I look, how I exercise, and almost all other aspects of my life. |
| I shouldn't have eaten that brownie. | Eating high-fat and high-sugar foods is problematic. It would be better if I didn't eat the brownie. However, I don't want to force myself to live with arbitrary rules ("shoulds"). If I eat a problematic food, I can monitor it and think of it as a problem to be solved. |

You can see the use of exaggerations and absolute-isms in this listing of irrational beliefs. Another method of categorizing irrational beliefs uses words and phrases to define seven different types of irrational thinking:

1. **Arbitrary inference.** Drawing a conclusion when evidence does not support the conclusion or is lacking entirely. "Since I didn't lose weight last week, I must be fooling myself to think I'm trying."

2. **Overgeneralization.** Creating a general rule from a single incident or observation. "I didn't walk very far today; I can't be serious about losing weight."

3. **Catastrophizing or magnification.** Exaggerating a problem or an event to make it seem hopeless or impossible to change. "I didn't lose weight last year; I can't do this."

4. **Cognitive deficiency.** Disregarding an important life situation. "I know I didn't exercise last week, but I can't believe I didn't lose weight."

5. **Dichotomous reasoning.** Believing that there are only two sides to an issue (good/bad, right/wrong) and no in-betweens. "I am either on a diet or off it."

6. **Oversocialization.** Failing to recognize and challenge the arbitrariness of many cultural mores. "I need liposuction to lose weight and a nose job to look decent. You can't be too thin."

7. **Negative thinking.** Focusing on aspects of behavior that you want to decrease and virtually excluding more positive thoughts. "I didn't exercise on three of seven days this week."

You may find the following Rational Emotive Therapy Worksheet and instructions of value in your efforts to persist at weight control. Try completing the worksheet by first writing out any stress reactions that you experienced recently under "consequences of accepting belief #1(C)."

If you felt angry or depressed or anxious or frustrated about something having to do with weight control, enter those emotional states under C. Then go back and try to identify the event that led to this emotional-reaction (A). Describe the belief that may have contributed to the emotional distress (B). Next, try using a disputing response similar to one in the previous examples (D). What effects does it have on you when you dispute your own irrational beliefs about weight control (E)?

**Instructions for completing RET worksheet:** Answer question C first. Then complete the remaining parts A through E.

A. **Activating event.** Describe the event you recently experienced in which you became upset. Example. "My friend told me I was a jerk."

B. **Irrational belief(s).** Describe the irrational belief(s) that you associate with this event and your becoming upset. Notice what was illogical in the belief by identifying extreme and absolute words in it. Example: "I must be worthless." The belief, "I am worthless" uses the extreme word "worthless."

C. **Consequences.** List an unpleasant emotional reaction you experienced recently. I could include feeling anxious, depressed, or some other unpleasant emotion. Think about any physical reactions you might have had (for example, stomach cramps, sweating, jittery-fidgeting, headache). Example: "I felt depressed."

D. **Disputing responses.** Write out questions, statements, and behaviors you engage in to dispute or refute your irrational belief. These are rational statements describing more appropriate ways of viewing the activating event. Example: "I would rather my friend did not call me a jerk. I guess I could have responded in a way that my friend would have preferred. I reacted badly in a particular situation; I wish I had acted more sensitively. I will try to remember that for the future."

E. **Effects.** Describe the effects on you of using disputing responses. These can include both changes in beliefs and changes in other unpleasant reactions to the activating event. Example: "I realize that I 'catastrophized' when my friend called me a jerk. I now believe that I would have preferred acting differently in the situation that led her to call me a jerk. I feel better, not as depressed anymore."

## Assertiveness

Can you recall your reaction to being belittled or taken advantage of, or in some way, interpersonally squashed or squelched? Frustrated, angry, anxious, and depressed feelings often follow such experiences. Expressing yourself openly, honestly, directly, and clearly can prevent those

---

## **Rational Emotive Therapy Worksheet**

A. Activating Event


B. Belief #1: Irrational belief:


C. Consequences of accepting belief #1:


D. Disputing responses to belief #1:


E. Effects of disputing belief #1:

---

unpleasant emotional effects. This type of communication lets others know you are a person who has rights—including the right to be treated kindly and respectfully.

Assertiveness is defined as any act that serves to maintain a person's rights; it is the open expression of preferences by words or actions in a manner that causes others to take them into account. When someone attempts to take advantage of you or treats you disrespectfully in some other way, you can react assertively, aggressively, or unassertively. Assertive behavior enhances your sense of self. It is expressive and it helps you feel good about yourself. It may or may not achieve the desired goal, however. Aggressiveness, by contrast, usually achieves desired goals by hurting or taking advantage of others. Aggressiveness is also expressive, but at the expense of other people. Unassertive behavior involves preventing yourself from standing up for your own rights. It often produces hurt, anxious, and angry feelings. It certainly fails to accomplish the goal of standing up for your rights.

Robert Alberti and Michael Emmons presented a "Universal Declaration of Human Rights" in their classic book on assertiveness, *Your Perfect Right*. This declaration of rights includes 30 articles or principles. Included among them are the right to think freely and the right to fair contracts in work and other transactions. You have the right to get what you pay for, to be treated respectfully, and to express yourself freely. If you express an opinion and get put down and discounted, your rights are being violated. When people attempt to take advantage of your time or talents, they are encroaching on your rights.

An example of a potential violation of rights that concerns weight controllers is ordering a meal prepared in a low-fat way in a restaurant and having the server refuse to comply with your wishes. When you make reasonable requests and those requests are agreed upon by the server, you certainly have the right to get what you pay for. Agreements at home with spouses and other family members also rely on respectful treatment. If your spouse agrees to eat potato chips and candy outside the house, you can justifiably become concerned when Milky Ways, M&Ms, and Pringles invade your kitchen cabinets. These situations sometimes lead to loud conflicts. Aggressive demands for change, met with resistance, produce interpersonal fireworks. An assertive approach is kinder and gentler. It states concerns directly and makes specific requests for change. It provides choice to the other person. The person may or may not respond in a desired fashion.

The key aspects of assertiveness include:

- **Eye contact.**  Look directly at another person when you are speaking to him or her. This effectively declares that you are sincere about what you are saying.

- **Body posture.**  The "weight" of your messages to others will be increased if you face the person, stand or sit appropriately close to him or her, lean toward him or her, and hold your head erect.

- **Gestures.**  A message accented with appropriate gestures takes on an added emphasis. Overenthusiastic gesturing, however, can be distracting.

- **Facial expression.**  Have you ever seen someone trying to express anger while smiling or laughing? It just doesn't come across. Effective assertions require an expression that agrees with the message.

- **Voice tone, inflection, volume.**  A whispered monotone will hardly convince another person that you mean business. A shouted epithet will bring a person's defenses into the path of communication. A level, well-modulated conversational statement can prove convincing without being intimidating.

- **Timing.**  Make spontaneous expression your goal. Hesitation may diminish the effect of an assertion. Judgment is necessary, however, to select an appropriate occasion. For example, speaking to your boss in front of a group of his or her subordinates may decrease his or her responsiveness to your request. Requesting a few quiet moments in a private office can promote acceptance of your assertion.

- **Content.** I saved this obvious dimension of assertiveness for last. Although *what* you say is clearly important, it is often less important than most people believe. A fundamental honesty in interpersonal communications and spontaneity of expression works best. That may mean saying forcefully, "I'm damn mad about what you just did!" rather than "You're an S.O.B.!" People who have, for years, hesitated because they "didn't know what to say" have found the practice of saying *something* to express their feelings at the time helps them communicate more effectively and comfortably.

Consider the example of the invasion of the junk food. Let's say the weight controller and spouse had agreed to ban such food from their house. The weight controller could angrily protest this "gross violation of our agreement." Resistance and hostility might flow from this exchange. In contrast, consider the likely reaction to, "Honey, I really have to struggle to control my eating. You recognized this six months ago when you agreed to ban junk food in the house. It upsets me to have this agreement violated. I would really appreciate it if you could get rid of the candy and chips tonight." Try delivering a message like this directly and forcefully, with appropriate eye contact and body language. Your spouse would not feel attacked. He or she might help you stay focused and enthusiastic. Your spouse may not comply with your request. However, he or she would probably remember the agreement and abide by it in the future. In any case, a loud, angry argument almost certainly would not emerge from this assertion.

## Effective Problem Solving

Five steps in effective problem solving include:

1. General orientation or "set"
2. Problem definition and formulation
3. Generation of alternatives
4. Decision making
5. Verification

Review the following definitions of these five steps and consider the examples related to weight control problems provided for each step.

### General Orientation or "Set"

The first step is to recognize that a problem exists and that you can try to cope with it. Problems are normal. Acting impulsively and giving up are not effective ways to deal with them. When a new problem develops or an old problem flares up, you can actively cope with the situation in a systematic fashion. Example: "My weight loss has slowed down and I am getting discouraged. I can cope with this problem, but I want to determine carefully what is wrong and develop a specific solution for it."

### Problem Definition and Formulation

As in phases of self-control, "defining the problem is half the solution." The best definitions of problems are concrete and specific rather than abstract and general. Include plenty of details (events, situations, circumstances, feelings, and so on) in your definitions. Try to separate relevant from irrelevant details. Help from others can prove useful during this step. Example: "Since my weight loss has slowed down, I must be eating more calories than I am burning up. Therefore, I need to reduce my caloric intake somehow or increase my exercising."

### Generation of Alternatives

This step suggests that you list several potential solutions before you try to evaluate or judge any of them (called "brainstorming"). Thinking of many alternatives increases the likelihood that you will come up with a good one. You may benefit from developing both specific and general solutions. Example: "I could cut out all desserts. I could start drinking my coffee black instead of with cream and sugar. I could increase my exercise level. I could try to switch to lower calorie meals."

### Decision Making

This step involves picking the best solution or strategy from the options described in the previous step. Try to anticipate the likely consequences of each of the alternative solutions you listed. Think of the personal and social consequences and the short- and long-term consequences of each alternative. Sometimes the best solution combines some of your alternatives. Perfect solutions do not exist. The best possible or "lessor of evils" solution could work well. Example: "I really like desserts occasionally and wouldn't realistically stop eating them forever. Also, I am too busy to increase my exercise level now. I think the best solution is to try to plan lower-calorie meals and also to gradually reduce the amount of cream and sugar in my coffee over the next month until I can drink it black. To help do this, I will start self-monitoring my coffee drinking and start planning menus one week in advance."

### Verification

This step involves trying out the chosen strategy to see if it works. Give the solution a fair chance—try it several times. It may take practice and several trials for you to make the solution effective. Keep track (probably in writing) of how well your solution worked. Have a concrete, specific definition of success so that you can really tell how well your solution worked. Defining the criterion for success in terms of something you can see and count is the best way to do this. If the solution you chose does not work, then recycle to steps (2) or (3) and try, try again. Example: "I'll try this strategy for one month. If I lose at least three pounds over the next month, then my strategy worked. If not, I'll go back to steps (2) and (3) and try again."

**Problem-solving worksheet.** Do you have a problem with your current eating and exercising patterns? Try using the following worksheet to begin solving it.

---

# Problem-Solving Worksheet

1. General orientation or "set": Recognize the existence of a problem.

2. Problem definition and formulation: Define the problem concretely and classify relevant information, issues, and goals.

3. Generation of alternatives: List the potential solutions or strategies for your problems.

4. Decision making: Choose the best solution or combination of solutions.

5. Verification: Try out the chosen strategy and see if it works. Record the results and any necessary modifications of the solution.

---

E. L. Edelstein and his colleagues provided a list of ten practices that they found "good copers" tended to do. These steps, from *Denial: A Clarification of Concepts and Research*, provide another useful way of summarizing effective problem solving.

1. They try to be as specific as possible about a problem.

2. They set a goal with realistic expectations.

3. They picture various intermediate steps that might help reach a feasible goal.

4. Then they act according to best judgment about the consequences.

5. In doing so, good copers acknowledge their emotional pressure points of vulnerability.

6. They keep a measure of emotional composure, because extremes tend to warp judgment.

7. They restrain themselves from undue, imaginary, or idealized possibilities in favor of practical and reachable goals.

8. There are usually a number of choices and options between black and white alternatives.

9. They find that denial is a useful temporary distraction and avoid self-pity, bitterness, or unwarranted optimism or pessimism.

10. They are ready to correct and monitor their own behavior, and seek guidance, knowing that belief in the capacity to cope competently fortifies morale and helps achieve good coping.

## Management of Sleep Problems

Most adults have difficulties getting adequate amounts of quality sleep occasionally. You may notice a weakening in your resolve when you feel tired. Exercising becomes much more difficult. Clarity in thinking about food choices wanes.

Consider using the following ideas and suggestions when sleeping becomes a problem.

### Assumptions

- Sleep is a natural biological state. Your body "wants to" sleep every night.

- Sometimes worries, anxieties, and related thoughts and feelings can overwhelm your body's natural inclination to sleep.

- If you can find effective methods of temporarily coping with concerns and refocusing your attention on your physical self, you will be able to sleep soundly.

- If you allow your bed to be a place where you grapple with everyday worries, your bed will become a stimulus associated with anxiety, not rest.

**Methods**

- Get out of bed if you are struggling to get to sleep for more than a few minutes.

- Attempt to formulate and write out a plan for coping with your concerns.

- After resolving your problem, albeit in a temporary and imperfect manner, begin relaxing by reading (avoid watching television—it's often too engrossing) or writing letters. Try using stretching, breathing, or progressive muscle relaxation exercises.

- When you begin to drift off to sleep, then—and only then—go back to bed.

- If these steps keep you awake longer than you like, realize that it is okay to be tired during the day sometimes. It won't hurt you that much to drag around for a day.

- Stay up to your usual bedtime before going to sleep. Also, get up at your usual time in the morning. In other words, don't sleep late to make up for the previous night.

- Try to increase your exercising on a regular basis and try to develop a consistent routine for relaxing each evening (for example, watch some TV, listen to music, read for a while). However, it is not helpful to force yourself to go to sleep at the same time each night. Just follow your routine in the evening and let yourself sleep when you are tired enough to drift off.

- Do not take either over-the-counter or prescription drugs to knock yourself out. These medicines do not induce the deep sleep that you need to feel rested. They produce, instead, a hangover of drowsiness, often accompanied by dry mouth, difficulty urinating, and confusion. The "benzodiazepines" (Halcion, Triazolam, Temazepam, Flurazepam) work better than antihistamines. But they produce such problems as "robound insomnia"—trouble sleeping once the medication is discontinued—and they can be habit-forming. Under no conditions does it make sense to take more than a single sleeping pill per week. If you can avoid taking drugs altogether, you will find the outcome much more satisfying.

# Key Principles

- Stressors are demands from the environment. Complex emotional responses resulting from experience with stressors are defined as stress.

- Hans Selye's General Adaptation Syndrome (GAS) suggests that people react to prolonged exposure to stressors in three stages. In the first stage ("alarm and mobilization"), physical resistance to stressors declines rapidly. The body reacts by becoming alert and tense, facilitating efforts to cope with the stressor. In stage two ("resistance"), powerful hormones (glucocorticoids) help the body maintain a high level of resistance. This resistance takes its toll in stage three ("exhaustion"). Severe anxiety, depression, nightmares, and physical weaknesses become apparent in this stage.

- Both major life events (such as moving, divorce, major changes in work) and much more minor daily hassles (such as interruptions, broken promises, losing something, traffic) can cause significant stress.

- Personality characteristics can affect how people manage stress. Type A people are hard-driving, energetic, and competitive. They tend to react with anger and hostility when confronting stressors. These personality characteristics make Type A people more likely to develop heart problems. In contrast, Type B characteristics include calmer reactions to stressors.

- Another adaptive style of responding to stressors is "hardiness." Hardier individuals respond to stressors more effectively. These individuals demonstrate *commitment* by approaching difficult life events with a sense of purpose. They see themselves *controlling* their lives by taking charge of stressors. Hardier individuals view stressors as *challenges* rather than problems to be endured. Weight controllers who grapple with stressors more actively and view them as challenges may be more likely to persist.

- Having good social support means having family and friends who provide emotional comforting, helpful information, and material goods when needed. Maintaining effective friendships and good connections with people can allow weight controllers to cope with the demands of their biologies in addition to the problems they face day to day.

- Stress inoculation includes an educational phase, a coping self-talk phase, a relaxation component, and a practice component. When faced with a stressor (like buying a new car or moving to a new city), it helps to ask questions about it, read about it, and take other steps to become educated about the stressor. Talking to yourself in a calming, focused manner can improve coping at critical moments. Developing relaxation skills through breathing exercises, progressive muscle relaxation, meditation, and other strategies can also help when confronting stressors. These techniques require practice in order to improve and master them.

- Stressors for weight controllers include such high-risk situations as getting home from work, watching TV, and holidays. High-risk situations are those in which you tend to have difficulties maintaining appropriate eating and exercising patterns. Some of these situations may seem perfectly normal to other people. The key is to identify situations that affect you in a problematic fashion. Weight controllers, who use a variety of coping responses to combat these high-risk situations are more likely to persist effectively in their weight control efforts. Coping responses include leaving the situation, calling or talking to someone, exercising, using low-calorie snacks, drinking non-caloric beverages, and self-monitoring.

- Another useful stress management procedure is the reattribution technique. People sometimes make problematic attributions about the causes of negative events. Attributions that suggest that the causes are internal, stable, and global can create depressed and anxious feelings. When a negative event occurs, it helps to make attributions that are *external* (finding factors other than yourself that contribute to them), *specific*, and *unstable* (suggesting the possibility of change over time).

- Rational Emotive Therapy (RET) techniques help people manage stress by changing irrational beliefs into more rational beliefs. Irrational beliefs include "absolute-isms" and exaggerations. When you use absolute-isms, you tell yourself that you have to, should, ought to, or must do certain things. These beliefs limit your sense of freedom. Exaggerations include beliefs that use such language as always, awful, essential, every, horrible, terrible, and totally. These beliefs exaggerate problems and contribute to a feeling of helplessness. When you find yourself using irrational beliefs, consider developing disputing responses to them. It also helps to examine the events that cause the use of such irrational beliefs. Types of irrational beliefs also include arbitrary inference, overgeneralization, catastrophizing or magnification, cognitive deficiency, dichotomous reasoning, oversocialization, and negative thinking.

- Assertiveness can help reduce stress. Assertiveness is defined as any act that serves to maintain your rights; it is the open expression of preferences by words or actions in a manner that causes others to take them into account. If you act unassertively, you fail to stand up for your own rights and often feel taken advantage of, hurt, or anxious. Aggressiveness might allow you to achieve your desired goals, but this comes at the expense of others. It may produce guilt or other negative reactions for you. Weight controllers find it useful to be assertive when others attempt to overfeed them or inhibit their exercising routines. Assertiveness includes looking directly at another person when speaking, talking calmly but forcefully, and using appropriate (direct) eye contact and body language.

- Another method of stress management involves the use of effective problem solving. Effective and active problem solving can diffuse the impact of stressors or manage their effects. Five steps in effective problem solving are general orientation or "set," problem definition and formulation, generation of alternatives, decision making, and verification. When weight controllers pay attention to these components, they produce more effective solutions to problems.

- The impact of stressors and feelings of stress can be magnified by lack of sleep. Since most adults experience some sleep problems occasionally, it may be helpful for you to understand how to get a good night's rest. First, some key assumptions include the notion that sleep is a natural biological state. Your body "wants to sleep" every night, but worries can prevent it from this natural inclination. It is critical to find methods of temporarily coping with concerns that keep you up at night. Some techniques that help people achieve restful sleep include getting out of bed if sleep becomes difficult. When out of bed, it helps to find a way to resolve a problem temporarily or to relax by reading or writing letters. After staying up one night, it is critical to stay up the following night until your usual bedtime. Over-the-counter and prescription drugs are not effective remedies. These medicines do not induce the deep sleep that you need to feel rested.

# Epilogue

"[People] are disturbed not by things, but by the view
which they take of them."

(Epictetus, first century, A.D.,
*The Enchiridion*)

"There's nothing either good or bad but thinking makes it so."

(William Shakespeare, *Hamlet*)

"A person's behavior springs from his ideas ... It is his attitude toward life which determines his relationship to the outside world."

(Alfred Adler, 1964, *Social Interest: A Challenge to Mankind*)

**Question:** How many workers are needed to change a light bulb in a burnout-prone environment?

**Answer:** At least nine.

- Two of whom did not make it to work today (one was sick, the other took a mental health day).

- One who was too hung over and another who was too depressed to notice that the bulb was out.

- Two who wouldn't do it because they were arguing over who did it the last time.

- Two who injured themselves trying to change the bulb too fast (one burned hand; one cut hand on the broken bulb).

- Finally, the bulb was replaced by an exasperated supervisor with high blood pressure, prior to her heart attack.

(Adapted from Whiton Paine, 1982, *Job Stress and Burnout*)

# 9

# Conclusions:
# Pathways to Persistence

A fundamental principle of weight loss and control is that for almost all people a lifelong commitment to a change in lifestyle, behavioral responses, and dietary practices is necessary.

(National Institutes of
Health, Technology
Assessment Conference
Statement, 1992)

## The Basic Plan

Do you have a "lifelong commitment" to persistence at weight control? Commitment provides the brick and mortar for change. As noted in Chapter 2, you cannot commit unless you make an active choice. Consider, again, your reaction to the following critical aspect of choosing to control your weight:

- **Truth 1 (from Chapter 2)** If you decide to lose weight, you are making a *choice*. You may choose to persist at weight control or you may choose not to lose weight. The decision is yours. This decision is not a moral or a religious one.

Cultural pressures, family members, and others may push you to lose weight. However, the biological barriers to weight control will keep you on the pathway you began before reading this book, unless you make the choice for long-term change. This choice only works well if you make it by yourself, for yourself, forever. External pushes and prods may lead to following the diet of the month, not to lifelong commitment. Recall the notion of weight control as a major athletic challenge. Just as all successful athletes demonstrate dedication and commitment in their training and thinking every day, so do successful weight controllers.

Perhaps your Decision Balance Sheet and other thoughts about weight control have helped you make a powerful commitment to change. This kind of commitment is reflected by the final two stages of change described in Chapter 3. As you review the following versions of those stages, consider: Are you there yet?

## Tentative Acceptance

This is a stage in which people settle in for the long haul. They experience a *peaceful sense of resolve* about weight control. They feel comfortable and have a clear direction for handling their challenging biologies. They also refine their knowledge of nutrition in this stage. Their understanding of the factors that affect weight control becomes clear, as well. They do struggle with their focusing or commitment sometimes. This happens quite often when they go on vacations or when their schedules are disrupted by illness or travel.

Weight controllers in this stage view exercise as either enjoyable or at least acceptable. They exercise very consistently. These weight controllers also consistently monitor their food and exercise. They assert themselves effectively in restaurants and other social situations regarding food. They prefer food to be prepared in a healthful way.

## Lifestyle Change

This stage describes the ultimate goal for weight controllers. Individuals in this difficult-to-reach stage seem *confident, but aggressively self-protective.* They are unwilling, and adamantly so, to place themselves in a position to become "mindless" again about their eating, exercising, and weight. They carefully observe their eating and exercising. They become very aware of changes in their moods, routines, relationships, work, and anything else that might trigger poor food choices or overeating. They feel confident about their knowledge of weight control—of what works and what does not. Eating and exercising patterns seem tied to emotions less than they used to be. When eating or exercising problems emerge, these individuals view these lapses as problems to be solved. They do not view problematic eating or exercising as weaknesses in their personalities or as reasons to give up. They also handle stressful situations directly without using food as a major method of coping. They actively seek healthful eating and exercising opportunities, even when traveling or vacationing.

Do the "peaceful sense of resolve" and "aggressive self-protectiveness" in these stages describe your current attitudes? If so, you are well on your way to persistence. Even weight controllers in these stages have plans for keeping their eating, exercising, and coping skills sharply focused and effective. You may find it useful to rethink your current long-term plan. The following version of the plan presented in Chapter 7 may prove helpful.

- **Step 1. Self-directed change: taking your best shot.** This may include adopting a low-fat eating plan such as the "Almost Never" plan or the Popcorn plan.

- **Step 2. Increase involvement of spouse and friends: getting a little help from your friends.** If step 1 does not produce positive results within a few weeks or months, you can involve others in your exercising program or your eating plan. Commitments are strengthened when they become more public.

- **Step 3. Join a reasonable weight control program: getting help from others with the same problem.** Both Take Off Pounds Sensibly (TOPS) and Weight Watchers can help some people, some of the time.

- **Step 4. Join a long-term professional program: getting help from professionals.** Hospitals and medical centers sometimes offer programs, such as Optifast, that can help more people more of the time than the nonprofessional programs listed in step 3. Look for programs conducted by psychologists with expertise in "cognitive-behavior therapy." Also, only programs that provide help for unlimited periods of time (no less than one year) are worth considering. Calls to local hospitals, colleges, and universities (psychology departments) may prove helpful. The following two national organizations have listings of psychologists in virtually every area of the United States: Association for Advancement of Behavior Therapy (212/279/7970) and American Psychological Association (202/336/5500).

The critical aspect of persistence in weight control is finding a way to nurture your commitment to it. This can occur only if you maintain practices such as weighing yourself at least weekly. Another aspect of commitment pertains to clothing. If your clothes get tighter, consider taking the necessary steps to activate the long-term plan. Simply having clothes enlarged or buying larger clothes can deactivate your plan and diminish commitment.

# Slumps and Slump-Busters

The *American Heritage Dictionary of the English Language* defines "slump" as follows:

**slump**. *int. v.* To fall or sink suddenly, as into a bog . . .
2. To decline suddenly; collapse. 3. To slide down suddenly.
4. To droop . . . - *n.* a sudden falling off or decline . . .

Batters slump. Pitchers slump. Golfers slump. Weight controllers also slump.

You can think of a slump as a very long lapse. Perhaps a slump lies somewhere between a lapse and a relapse. Regardless of terminology, almost all weight controllers know the experience. Very few people, if any, go from having major weight problems into Lifestyle Change without encountering some serious bumps along the way.

The preceding chapters describe many of the factors that can cause slumps and some potential solutions to them. This section presents some new ideas and some new versions of the ideas from previous chapters. You can think of these ideas and suggestions as slump-busters. They could help you reactivate your commitment to persistence at weight control when slumps slow you down.

## *Help From Your Friends*

Have you wondered why smokers who have quit for months, or sometimes years, begin lighting up again? Or, why do reformed alcoholics start drinking again after leading a sober life for weeks, months, or years? Research by Alan Marlatt and many other behavioral scientists shows that conflicts between people often lead to such relapses. Consider Judy's story in the following case history as an example of the power of problems in relationships.

---

### Case History: Judy Battles with Bob— and Then Food

Judy and Bob had been married for four tumuluous years. Judy was a successful journalist for a major newspaper and Bob was an accountant at a large firm in the same city. They both had busy professional lives filled with demands and challenges. They often devoted more time to their professions than their relationship. They seemed to fight about almost everything, and food was no exception.

Judy decided to work conscientiously to improve her eating and exercising habits. She was approximately 40 pounds overweight when she began this self-directed quest. Bob was also somewhat overweight, but he did not want to make it a priority in his life. When Judy began eating lower-fat foods and making more and more time for exercising, Bob objected. They began fighting about what to eat and, more specifically, about what Judy should eat. After several weeks of these skirmishes, Judy laid down the law to Bob. "I'm going to decide what I eat, and you must learn to live with it. If I want your ideas about it, I'll ask. Otherwise, this is important to me, and I want you to let me make these changes." Bob conceded Judy's right to manage her own body. The skirmishes decreased and a peaceful, although somewhat uneasy, state emerged.

Over the course of the next year, Judy lost almost all of the weight she wanted to lose and became a committed exerciser. She used her health club membership very effectively. She found that exercising provided a good outlet for her stressful life. Judy often talked to Bob about this and encouraged him to consider using this facility to help himself, as well. Bob resisted and never accompanied Judy to the club.

One day Judy discovered that Bob had an affair with a woman at his office. Judy's relationship with Bob had never been great, but it had become something of a comfortable alternative to loneliness. Now all that changed. Judy saw this violation of their commitment to each other as a major assault. She and Bob argued and fought with an intensity she never knew she had within her. During this time, food and exercising became "unimportant" to Judy, "Nothing else mattered. I just didn't care."She ate what was available, and she "just didn't feel like" exercising anymore. It didn't take long for the weight to come back on and for the old habits to reemerge in full force.

Perhaps your conflicts with important people in your life have been less dramatic than Judy and Bob's. Even minor disagreements between couples can produce critical lapses. In addition, many spouses try to meddle too much in the life of the weight controller. They may see the weight controller eating high-fat foods. They may notice the weight controller decrease his or her frequency of exercising for a few days or a week. When family members use these observations to pressure the weight controller to get back on track, this usually backfires. "I'll show you!" can become a terrific motivator for eating cookies and ice cream.

Because many families have problems with meddling, interfering, or trying to "help too much," I developed the following guidelines for spouses and family members. You may find it useful to photocopy this next section to give to your spouse or family members. The information provides gentle reminders of how to help without interfering.

## Supporting a Person's Weight Control Efforts

Losing weight and keeping it off is a very difficult process. You can make it easier for your spouse, friend, or partner. Here are several suggestions to help you support and encourage someone you know who is trying to control his or her weight.

- **General attitude toward a person's weight control effort**

    1. *Be positive*—Convey to the weight controller that even though it is very difficult to control weight, you believe he or she can do it with a lot of hard work and concentration. This attitude will boost the person's self-confidence in weight control while acknowledging the difficulties of it. Avoid negative comments, criticism, and coercion. These are unhelpful and demoralizing, and will engender negative feelings between you and the weight controller. As a result, they may decrease the weight controller's motivation to continue his or her efforts. This, in turn, could cause him or her to eat more—not less—and thwart the likelihood of success in the long run.

    2. *Be reinforcing*—acknowledge the weight controller's accomplishments. Compliments, attention, encouragement, and tangible reinforcement in response to the weight controller's efforts will help him or her stay motivated and adhere to the plan. Remember, be sincere; superficiality will be interpreted as condescending and aversive.

    3. *Be realistic*—Weight control requires tremendous effort and skill to overcome strong biological forces. People who are trying to lose weight must adopt eating and exercising patterns that are much more stringent than those engaged in by individuals who do not have a weight problem. Don't expect the weight controller to be perfect, or even close to perfect. Occasional slips of overeating, inactivity, weight gain, and failure to adhere to plans will occur. Help the weight controller learn from these experiences rather than dwell on them as "failures."

    4. *Communicate*—Occasionally inquire about the weight controller's progress. Ask him or her how you can help, thereby complimenting the weight controller's individual efforts. Be open to discussing the realistic trials and tribulations of weight control and to assist in problem-solving difficulties or in sharing successes.

- **Helping a person change his or her eating habits**

    1. Limit the amount of fattening foods in the weight controller's presence (for example, avoid eating fatty and sugary foods in front of the weight controller; keep fattening items out of your home or away from the office).

2. Increase the amount of nutritious, low-fat foods available to the weight controller.

3. Do not encourage the weight controller to eat foods he or she is trying to limit or avoid (for example, refrain from saying, "Let's go out for ice cream," or "Oh, come on, a little bit isn't going to hurt you.").

4. Help the weight controller prepare foods and recipes in a low-fat way. Encourage experimentation and adventure.

5. Adopt appropriate eating habits (for example, not eating when full, eating appropriate portions, eating in a slow, deliberate fashion, eating regularly or on a schedule, limiting snacking, limiting the number of eating situations). You may not have a weight problem, but better eating habits may improve your health and will support the weight controller's efforts.

6. Plan activities with the weight controller that do not revolve solely around food (for example, sports events, concerts, games).

7. When you go to a restaurant with the weight controller, select places that make low-fat/low-sugar eating as pleasant as possible.

- **Helping a person change his or her exercise habits**

    1. Plan activities with the weight controller that involve exercise (for example, walking, hiking, sports activities).

    2. Become an exercise partner. You will reap the same physical benefits as your partner.

    3. Support and encourage the weight controller's individual efforts to exercise.

## Health Clubs and Trainers

Many years ago health clubs were places for fanatics, weight lifters, grunters and groaners, and athletes. Now they serve as a social melting pot and meeting place. They also provide many comforts and a very wide range of activities, including low-impact and no-impact aerobics classes, water aerobics activities, yoga, instruction in almost every indoor sport imaginable, and machines, machines, machines. These centers of physical activity can serve as effective slump-busters. When people join such centers, they tend to use them, at least for a while. Their novelty and diversity of activities can motivate refocusing on healthy eating and exercising.

When selecting a health club, keep in mind their three most important qualities: location, location, location! You will find that you actually use your health club when you either live very near it or work near it. If you belong to a health club located close to your house, you may use it in the morning. Almost all of the hundreds (perhaps thousands) of weight controllers with whom I have worked over the last 20 years, and who have succeeded at this difficult enterprise, have exercised primarily in the morning. Morning exercise proves most reliable because it interferes less in your daily life. After all, in the morning, you have complete control of your schedule and you can exercise before getting showered and dressed for the day. Exercising at any other time of the day requires taking a second shower and interrupting activities. Yet another advantage of morning exercise concerns attitude. You may have noticed that you feel better during the day if you exercise first thing in the morning. For all of these reasons, consider choosing a health club near your home, if at all possible.

Many people have used trainers to help motivate them. Working with a trainer can help you learn about different types of equipment. For example, if you decide to begin a weight lifting program, a trainer could provide important instruction on technique and help you set up an effective regimen. Trainers can also help motivate you. They provide encouragement and support. Also, if you set up an appointment with a trainer, and particularly if you prepay for that appointment, you greatly increase your chances of doing some constructive exercising that day.

Try to find trainers who have advanced degrees in physical education or who are certified as athletic trainers (A.T.C.). The American College of Sports Medicine also certifies trainers. If you select a trainer who has an advanced degree in physical education or appropriate certification, you can feel more confident that the advice you get is grounded in science rather than hearsay. Unfortunately, personal trainers can cost anywhere from $10 to $100 per hour. Prices vary depending on standards used within the health club, training, and whether the trainers come to your house or you go to their facility. If you are in a major slump and can find no other way out of it, the price of weekly sessions with a personal trainer for a month or two may well be worth it.

## Equipment

"I couldn't get myself focused until I bought a treadmill. It was a major expense (almost $2000), but I get on that thing every day now. I really like it. I like having it in my house because of the flexibility it provides and the reminder it provides. When I see it sitting there (which is very easy because it's huge), I know how important my weight control efforts are to me." These sentiments were expressed by one of my former clients. She had indeed gotten into a major slump and was very excited about the way her new treadmill helped her get out of it.

An equipment purchase can prove very motivating for the reasons this former client outlined. Having the equipment in your home makes it much easier to exercise. Many people who have weight problems are reluctant to go to a health club. They find the looks and comments of other people disconcerting. Of course, overweight people have as much right to use facilities at health clubs as any other customers. Yet the feelings can be so strong for some people that overcoming them is very difficult. Some people also live in climates that make outside exercising, such as walking or jogging, particularly challenging. These challenges can also be overcome with appropriate clothing. However, some people remain reluctant to exercise outside of their homes.

If you find yourself in a slump and believe that you may increase your exercising with the purchase of a piece of equipment, consider doing just that. Some very adequate exercycles are available for a few hundred dollars. More elaborate pieces of equipment, such as treadmills, carry much higher price tags. The best way to decide which piece of equipment makes the most sense for you is to go to a health club and try out the equipment. If you try out various pieces of equipment for several weeks, you will determine which kind is most comfortable for you and which you would be most likely to use consistently. *Consumer Reports* routinely evaluates exercise equipment for home use. Your local library includes copies of recent issues of *Consumer Reports*. The publisher of this magazine also prints books that summarize major findings on an annual basis. Before spending hundreds of dollars, perhaps thousands, it makes sense to examine the available evidence about which pieces of equipment work most effectively and reliably.

## Self-Help Programs and Books

The long-term plan presented earlier in this chapter includes the possibility of participating in either TOPS or Weight Watchers. These programs cost either nothing (TOPS) or relatively modest amounts of money (Weight Watchers). Certainly every major city in the United States and many smaller towns have TOPS and Weight Watchers groups that meet quite frequently. These approaches provide support for change and may help you focus at a time when nothing else seems to work. These self-help programs, as well as professional programs, can serve as effective slump-busters.

The publisher of this book, New Harbinger Publications, publishes a variety of self-help books and tapes that can help you refocus. For example, among New Harbinger's titles that you might find helpful are: *Body Relaxed—Mind at Ease, Self-Esteem, The Relaxation & Stress Reduction Workbook, Risk-Taking for Personal Growth, Thoughts & Feelings: The Art of Cognitive Stress Intervention*, and *The New Three Minute Mediator*. Several other publishers produce materials on relaxation, eating, nutrition, depression, and other topics that may reawaken your commitment to effective weight control. New Harbinger Publication's books and tapes can be ordered by calling 1/800/748-6273. Many other publications like these are widely available at all bookstores. The bibliography at the end of this book includes other titles on the topics of exercise, weight control, nutrition, and stress management.

## Radical Changes in Diet

Chapter 5 included a variety of eating plans. If you have been following one of those plans, consider switching to a different one. For example, if you follow the Self-Monitoring plan, you may notice a tremendous increase in your ability to focus and change your behaviors. The Popcorn plan, Vegetarian plan, and Very low-calorie diets (VLCDs) offer additional possibilities. When considering the use of a VLCD, appropriate medical and behavioral supervision are highly recommended. As noted in Chapter 5, Optifast programs offer among the best of the available hospital-based treatment approaches that incorporate a liquid VLCD.

Radical changes in diets can sometimes help break slumps. They require concentration and may serve as rallying points for change. Usually, radical dietary approaches suffer the same fate as all diets: They do not work for very long. But as a temporary step, making a major shift in your eating plan could spark important changes.

## Medications

Physicians began prescribing amphetamines (Benzedrine) more than 50 years ago to help people lose weight. Unfortunately, not only does Benzedrine reduce appetite, it is an addictive drug that produces a "high" that people crave. Thousands of people became addicted to Benzedrine in an attempt to lose weight. That drug and others like it can no longer be prescribed in the United States or England for weight control. Prescriptions for those drugs are carefully monitored by governments.

Many physicians know this sad tale. They believe that any drug prescribed for weight control may cause unnecessary harm—more harm than good. This view, while understandable, no longer fits the current scientific information about medications for weight control. Despite the bias against them, some modern medications can help people decrease their appetite and feel full sooner. These efforts can occur with virtually no risk for causing addictions. Does this sound too good to be true? Well, the story is more complicated than this.

Medications that help control appetite also can produce such side effects as depression, irritability, dizziness, insomnia, and nausea. The best of the medications produce very few of these effects for most people. However, these effects, when they occur, can be quite annoying. Also, the research on these medications suggests that they work well while they are taken. However, soon after people stop taking them, even if they have taken them for six months or one year, many people regain all the weight they lost. Also, most people seem to lose only relatively small amounts of weight on these medications.

Modern medications for weight control still have an important role to play. First, if you take these medications while participating in an active weight control program, their benefits may be better than those that have appeared in the scientific literature thus far. In other words, relatively few studies of the use of modern medications with ongoing treatment for weight control have appeared. It seems likely that taking medications when involved in a professional treatment program may prove to be an effective slump-buster. I have seen this happen with many of my clients. Their weight losses slowed down or stopped for various reasons. After they began a course of drug treatment, their eating and exercising improved markedly. I have seen quite a few people use the medications, lose 10 to 20 pounds, get off the medications, and continue to lose weight.

Two specific medications have the best scientific basis for their use and are available in the United States. It makes sense to take both of these medications at the same time because they have different effects. First, phentermine (trade name, Ionamin) decreases appetite. It has mild stimulant properties, but people do not become addicted to it. Fifteen to 30 milligrams of Ionamin can be taken daily to decrease appetite. When phentermine or Ionamin is taken along with fenfluramine (trade name, Pondamin), the effects seem most powerful and produce the fewest side effects. Fenfluramine blocks the release of a certain chemical in the brain (serotonin). This action makes you feel full much sooner during the course of a meal than you would feel without taking the drug. If you take Ionamin and Pondamin together, you have less desire to eat due to the Ionamin, and you feel fuller sooner due to the Pondamin. The dose for Pondamin goes up to 60 milligrams daily.

It is critical to emphasize that it only makes sense to take these medications if you are participating in a professionally conducted weight control program. For example, Pondamin may cause symptoms of depression. Abruptly withdrawing from Pondamin can also create depressed feelings. In a professional weight control program, these effects can be anticipated and handled appropriately. Also, the scientific research suggests that these medications would produce few benefits unless weight controllers get help focusing on eating and exercising through a professional program while they are taking the medications.

If prescription medications for weight control can help some participants in professional programs, can over-the-counter drugs (such as Dexatrim and others) help anyone? Probably not. Frank Greenway, a UCLA nutritionist, recently reviewed the research on the two nonprescription drugs that are available in the United States, phenylpropanolamine (PPA) and benzocaine. PPA works like Ionamin; it acts as a mild stimulant. But it does not work as well as Ionamin. PPA can produce some small weight losses, but the effects do not last long. PPA is found in most nonprescription "weight control" drugs. Benzocaine is found in some over-the-counter "appetite" or "weight control" drugs. It supposedly numbs the taste, smell, or other qualities of food. It does not work at all. If you want to try medications for weight control, first join a professional program. Then discuss this possibility with your therapist and consider only prescription medications—if you and your therapist view that option as worthwhile.

## Balance in Life

"I had lost 30 pounds and had kept it off for two years. Then I started having major conflicts in my job. I felt trapped and had nowhere to go. My field is very overcrowded and a job as good as mine is very hard to find. I began withdrawing from people both at work and in the rest of my life. Since I am single, this meant I was spending more and more time alone. I began eating more, taking comfort in food again, and gaining weight."

I have seen a version of this story many times. Weight controllers who find their lives becoming imbalanced often get into lapses, slumps, or relapses. Too much time on your hands or not enough time for fun can lead to giving in to your biology. Your fat cells and other biological systems are always knocking on your door asking for attention. If your life becomes less distracting or more unpleasant, the knock on the door gets louder and louder. Feeding the fat cells also provides a very powerful, immediate form of comfort and enjoyment. You can certainly understand the power of that form of relaxation and comfort. Every weight controller can relate to this.

When you find yourself in a slump, consider trying to regain balance by looking at the quality of your social life. How are your relationships at work? How is your social life outside of work? Can you find some way to become reenergized about people both at work and at home? This could involve joining a new group or club after work. It could also involve taking up a new hobby that includes other people. Finding people at work to talk to and changing the nature of your job may help as well. Weight control exists in the context of your social world. Weight controllers do not simply eat and exercise. Eating and exercising takes place within families, work environments, and other critical social relationships. When those contexts become dysfunctional, weight control becomes dysfunctional.

You can sometimes identify signs of imbalance in your life by the way you think and talk about food. Do you describe your affection for food in glowing terms? Some of my clients say things like, "I love, love, love fresh strawberries." Strawberries, broccoli, cookies, and other foods can substitute in this sentence. Can you really *love* food? Isn't love supposed to be a special emotion shared by people with each other? If you hear yourself thinking in such terms of endearment toward fruits, vegetables, desserts, or any food, take a look at the balance in your life. Try to find ways in which you can improve your relationships with people and your contact with people.

## Psychotherapy

According to the *Diagnostic and Statistical Manual of Mental Disorders*, a "major depressive syndrome" includes at least five of the following symptoms that are present for at least two weeks and show a change from previous functioning. At least one of the symptoms must be either (1) depressed mood or (2) loss of interest in pleasure.

1. Depressed mood ... most of the day, nearly every day ...

2. Markedly [decreased] interest or pleasure in all, or almost all, activities most of the day, nearly every day ...

3. Significant weight loss or weight gain when not dieting ... or increase in appetite nearly every day ...

4. Insomnia or hypersomnia [excess sleeping] nearly every day

5. [Excess physical movement or slowing down in physical movements] nearly every day

6. Fatigue or loss of energy every day

7. Feelings of worthlessness or excessive or inappropriate guilt ... nearly every day

8. [Decreased] ability to think or concentrate, or indecisiveness, nearly every day ...

9. Recurrent thoughts of death (not just fear of dying), recurrent suicidal [thoughts] without a specific plan or suicide attempt or specific plan for committing suicide.

Many people experience significant depressions and other forms of psychological distress at some points in their lives. You can see how a major depressive syndrome can interfere with successful weight control. When feeling depressed, people struggle to stay focused on almost anything in their lives, let alone something as difficult as warding off the biology of excess weight gain. I have heard many people say, "I just didn't care." This statement often accompanies significant lapses or slumps. Unfortunately, once again, your biology has no sympathy. If you feel lousy, for whatever reason, your biology seems more than happy to add excess pounds.

People try many things to get out of depression and other unpleasant psychological states. You can try talking to close friends, taking vacations, or changing something significant in your life. When all of your best efforts do not produce positive change, consider taking the next step. You can seek professional help for marital problems or problems with your moods, such as depression. You can ask close friends or relatives for referrals to licensed professionals in your area whom they know or have heard good things about. You can also call your local hospital or university and ask how to get professional assistance.

Most health insurance policies cover substantial amounts of the costs involved with such treatment. Most communities also provide relatively low-cost counseling. You can find these services by calling your church or synagogue or your local mental health association.

If at all possible, try to find a therapist who is licensed in your state and either a psychologist, social worker, or psychiatrist. Psychologists receive five to eight years of training beyond a bachelor's degree. This training focuses on the scientific aspects of helping people change. Social workers receive one to three years of training beyond a bachelor's degree, focused on how to form good relationships with people and to understand resources available in communities that can prove helpful. Psychiatrists receive a medical degree and then several years of training beyond that to help them specialize in how to help people with significant problems in their lives. Psychiatrists are the only mental health professionals who can prescribe medications. However, this may not be an advantage. In my opinion, most psychiatrists prescribe medications too quickly. You can find yourself being treated with a serious and powerful set of medications (with sometimes complicated side effects) while other, less chemical, methods can produce better outcomes. I, therefore, recommend seeing a licensed psychologist or social worker before seeing a psychiatrist. If medications seem like they would be helpful to you, these other licensed mental health professionals will certainly recommend that you get a consultation from a psychiatrist in order to use such treatments. I believe that if you can find a way of changing without using medications, it is the best thing to do.

Many weight controllers who become depressed delay getting help. Certainly problems take a while to resolve on your own. You may ask friends or family for help. You may read about the problem and attempt to change yourself. These efforts are worthy of admiration and respect. If and when they do not produce positive outcomes, however, please take action quickly. Your biology acts very quickly to cause you trouble. A lapse quickly turns into a slump or a relapse. To avoid this downward spiral, *action* must become your middle name. Your biology does not allow you to stay in a slump very long without punishing you much more severely than the person who doesn't struggle with weight problems.

Sport psychologists provide very similar advice to professional and other elite athletes. When athletes struggle with emotional issues, their performance declines, just as your weight increases. Performance declines can rapidly become major slumps. Major slumps can ruin careers. Athletes, and weight controllers, must take action quickly to grapple with whatever problems face them. Quick actions on the part of athletes can end slumps. The same applies to you.

# Key Principles

- Remember, from Chapter 2, if you decide to lose weight, you are making a *choice*. You may choose to persist at weight control or you may choose not to lose weight. The decision is yours. This decision is not a moral or religious one.

- Weight control is a major athletic challenge (as noted in Chapter 2). Just as all successful athletes demonstrate dedication and commitment in their training and thinking every day, so do successful weight controllers.

- Highly committed and persistent weight controllers frequently experience a "peaceful sense of resolve" and "aggressive self-protectiveness" as attitudes toward their weight control (from Chapter 3).

- A long-term plan for successful weight control could include self-directed change; increased involvement of spouse and friends; and joining a reasonable weight control program.

- Almost all weight controllers experience lapses, slumps, or re-lapses. Various slump-busters encourage weight controllers to take action quickly to reverse the pattern that led to the slump.

- Potential slump-busters include getting better help from friends and family; trying health clubs and/or trainers; purchasing at-home exercise equipment; reading self-help books and trying self-help programs (such as TOPS or Weight Watchers); making radical (but reasonable) changes in diet; trying the modern medications for weight control—only while participating in a professionally conducted weight control program; seeking better balance in one's life (particularly by increasing the quality of one's social life both at work and at home); and obtaining psychotherapy from a licensed mental health professional if problems become particularly severe.

# Epilogue

"... let us run with endurance the race that is set before us ... "

(Hebrews 12:1)

# Bibliography

I encourage you to read about nutrition, exercise, and weight control to support and reinforce your persistence. The books are listed in four categories: exercise, nutrition, stress management, and weight control. They include many that are easily read by most people with high school or college educations. Those marked with asterisks are more technically oriented and were written especially for health care professionals. You may wish to try both nontechnical and more technically oriented books to see what kind of information is available.

## Exercise

Blair, S.N. (1991). *Living with exercise.* Dallas, TX: American Health Publishing Co. (telephone: 800/736/7323).

Blair, S.N. (1991). Weight loss through physical activity. *Weight Control Digest, 1,* 17, 20-24.

Curless, M.R. (1992). Only the fit stay young. *Self,* September, pp. 180-181.

*Dishman, R.K. (Ed.). (1988). *Exercise adherence: Its impact on public health.* Champaign, IL: Human Kinetics Publishers (telephone: 800/747/4457).

Euloff, N., and Thomas, D.O. (1987, April). Exercise videos: A critical analysis. *Fitness in Business,* pp. 179-183.

Exercise bicycles. (1990, November). *Consumer Reports,* pp. 746-757.

Galvin, J. (1992). *The exercise habit: Your personal road map to developing a lifelong exercise commitment.* Champaign, IL: Human Kinetics Publishers.

*Heil, J. (1993). *Psychology of sport injury.* Champaign, IL: Human Kinetics Publishers.

*Horn, T.S. (Ed.). (1992). *Advances in sport psychology.* Champaign, IL: Human Kinetics Publishers

*Kendzierski, D., and Johnson, W. (1993). Excuses, excuses, excuses: A cognitive behavioral approach to exercise implementation. *Journal of Sport and Exercise Psychology, 15*, 207-219.

Kusinitz, I., Fine, M., and Editors of Consumer Reports Books. (1983). *Physical fitness for practically everybody: The consumer's union report on exercise.* Mount Vernon: NY: Consumers Union.

Latella, F.S., Conkling, W., and Editors of Consumers Reports Books. (1989). *Get in shape stay in shape.* NY: Consumer Reports Books.

Morgan, W.P. (1978). The mind of a marathoner. *Psychology Today, 11*, 38-49.

Orlick, T. (1990). *In pursuit of excellence: How to win in sport and life through mental training* (2nd ed.). Champaign, IL: Human Kinetics Publishers

Rippe, J.M., and Amend, P. (1992). *The exercise exchange program.* NY: Simon & Schuster.

*Silva, J.M. III, and Weinberg, R.S. (Eds.). (1984). *Psychological foundations of sport.* Champaign, IL: Human Kinetics Publishers

Thayer, R.E. (1987). Energy, tiredness, and tension effects of a sugar snack versus moderate exercise. *Journal of Personality and Social Psychology, 52*, 119-125.

Vanltallie, T.B., and Hadley, L. (1988). *The best spas.* NY: Harper & Row.

# Nutrition

Are you eating right? (1992, October) *Consumer Reports*, pp. 644-655.

Bailey, C., and Bishop, L. (1989). *The fit-or-fat woman.* Boston: Houghton-Mifflin Company.

*Blass, E. (1989). Opioids, sweets, and a mechanism for positive affect: Broad motivational implications. In J. Dobbing (Ed.) *Sweetness.* NY: Springer-Verlag.

Bloom, M. (1989). What's good on the menu? *Chicago* magazine.

Brody, J. (1987). *Jane Brody's nutrition book.* NY: Bantam Books.

Cohler, S. (1988). Food for thought. *Psychology Today*, p. 30.

*Dobbing, J. (Ed.). (1987). *Sweetness.* NY: Springer-Verlag.

Eisenman, P.A., Johnson, S.C., and Benson, J.E. (1990). *Coaches guide to nutrition and weight control* (2nd ed.). Champaign, IL: Human Kinetics Publishers (telephone: 800/747/4457).

Feiden, M. (1989). *The calorie factor: The dieter's companion.* NY: Simon & Schuster.

Florman, Monte, Florman, Marjorie, and Editors of Consumer Reports. (1990). *Fast foods: Eating in and eating out.* NY: Consumer Reports Books.

Nager, Victoria, and Nager, Valerie. (1989). *Dining lite Chicago.* Chicago: Brooke-Brandon Communications Co.

Natow, A.B., and Heslon, J. (1989). *The fat counter.* NY: Pocket Books.

Netzer, C.T. (1991). *The complete book of food counts* (2nd ed.). NY: Dell Publishing.

Scanlon, D., and Strauss, L. (1992). *Diets that work: For weight control or medical needs.* Los Angeles: Lowell House.

Sims, E.A.H. (1974). Studies in human hyperphagia. In G. Bray and J. Bethune (Eds.). *Treatment and management of obesity.* New York: Harper & Row.

Sims, E.A.H., Danforth, E., et al. (1973). Endocrine and metabolic effects of experimental obesity in man. *Recent Progress in Hormone Research, 29,* 457-487.

Warshaw, H.S. (1990). *The restaurant companion: A guide to healthier eating out.* Chicago: Surrey Books.

# Stress Management

*Adler, A. (1964). *Social interest: A challenge to mankind.* New York: Capricorn Books.

Alberti, R.E., and Emmons, M.L. (1990). *Your perfect right: A guide to assertive living* (6th ed.). San Luis Obispo, CA: Impact Publishers.

*American Psychiatric Association. (1987). *Diagnostic and statistical manual of mental disorders* (3rd ed. rev.). Washington, D.C.

Barlow, D.H., and Rapee, R.M. (1991). *Mastering stress: A lifestyle approach.* Dallas: American Health Publishing Company (telephone: 800/736/7323).

*Bernstein, D.A., and Borkovec, D.T. (1973). *Progressive relaxation training: A manual for the helping professions.* Champaign, IL: Research Press.

Birkedahl, N. (1991). *Older & wiser: A workbook for coping with aging.* Oakland, CA: New Harbinger Publications, Inc.

Blevins, W. (1993). *Your family / yourself.* Oakland, CA: New Harbinger Publications, Inc.

Bourne, E.J. (1990). *The anxiety and phobia workbook.* Oakland, CA: New Harbinger Publications, Inc.

Burns, D.E. (1989). *The feeling good handbook: Using the new mood therapy in everyday life.* NY: William Morrow & Company.

Catalano, M.E. (1987). *The chronic pain control workbook.* Oakland, CA: New Harbinger Publications, Inc.

Catalano, E., with Webb, W., Walsh, J., and Morin, C. (1990). *Getting to sleep.* Oakland, CA: New Harbinger Publications, Inc.

Cautela, J.R., and Groden, J. (1991). *Relaxation: A comprehensive manual for adults, children, and children with special needs.* Champaign, IL: Research Press.

Copeland, M.E., with McKay, M. (1992). *The depression workbook.* Oakland, CA: New Harbinger Publications, Inc.

Davis, M., Eshelman, E.R., and McKay, M. (1988). *The relaxation & stress reduction workbook* (3rd ed.). Oakland, CA: New Harbinger Publications, Inc.

*Dworkin, S.F., Chen, A.C.N., Schubert, M.M., and Clark, D.W. (1984). Cognitive modification of pain: Information in combination with $N_2O$. *Pain, 19,* 339-351.

*Edelstein, E.L., Nathanson, D.L., and Stone, A.M. (1989). *Denial: A clarification of concepts and research.* New York: Plenum Press.

Ellis, A., and Harper, R.A. (1975). *A new guide to rational living.* Hollywood, CA: Wilshire Book Co.

Fanning, P. (1988). *Visualization for change.* Oakland, CA: New Harbinger Publications, Inc.

Fanning, P., and McKay, M. (1993). *Being a man.* Oakland, CA: New Harbinger Publications, Inc.

Grasha, A.F., and Kirschenbaum, D.S. (1986). *Adjustment and competence: Concepts and applications*. Minneapolis: West Publishing Company.

Harp, D., with Feldman, N. (1990). *The new three minute meditator*. Oakland, CA: New Harbinger Publications, Inc.

Holmes, T.H., and Rahe, R.H. (1967). The social readjustment rating scale. *Journal of Psychosomatic Research, 11,* 216.

Jacobson, E. (1929). *Progressive relaxation*. Chicago: University of Chicago Press.

Kane, J. (1991). *Be sick well: A healthy approach to chronic illness*. Oakland, CA: New Harbinger Publications, Inc.

*Kanfer, F.H., and Goldstein, A.P. (Eds.). (1991). *Helping people change: A textbook of methods* (4th ed.). NY: Pergamon Press.

*Kanfer, F.H., and Schefft, B.K. (1988). *Guiding the process of therapeutic change*. Champaign, IL: Research Press.

Kirkland, K., and Hollandsworth, J.G., Jr. (1980). Effective test-taking: Skills acquisition versus anxiety-reduction techniques. *Journal of Consulting and Clinical Psychology, 48,* 431-439.

Klarreich, S.H. (1990). *Work without stress: A practical guide to emotional well-being on the job*. NY: Brunner/Mazel.

*Lazarus, R.S., and Folkman, S. (1984). *Stress, appraisal, and coping*. New York: Springer.

Lecker, S. (1978). *The natural way to stress control*. New York: Grosset & Dunlap.

Lewinsohn, P.M., Munoz, R.F., Youngren, M.A., and Szeiss, A.M. (1986). *Control your depression* (rev.). NY: Prentice-Hall Press.

Marks, I.M. (1978). *Living with fear: Understanding and coping with anxiety*. NY: McGraw-Hill.

Markway, B.G., Carmin, C.N., Pollard, C.A., and Flynn, T. (1992). *Dying of embarrassment: Help for social anxiety and social phobia*. Oakland, CA: New Harbinger Publications, Inc.

Martin, R.A., and Poland, E.Y. (1980). *Learning to change: A self-management approach to adjustment*. NY: McGraw-Hill.

McKay, M., and Fanning, P. (1993). *Time out from stress* (two ten-minute cassettes). Oakland, CA: New Harbinger Publications, Inc.

McKay, M., and Fanning, P. (1993) *Self-Esteem* (2nd ed.). Oakland, CA: New Harbinger Publications, Inc.

McKay, M., and Fanning, P. (1991). *Prisoners of belief: Exposing and changing beliefs that control you life*. Oakland, CA: New Harbinger Publications, Inc.

McKay, M., Davis, M., and Fanning, P. (1981). *Thoughts & feelings: The art of stress intervention*. Oakland, CA: New Harbinger Publications, Inc.

McKay, M., Davis, M., and Fanning, P. (1983). *Messages: The communication skills book*. Oakland, CA: New Harbinger Publications, Inc.

McKay, M., Rogers, P.D., and McKay, J. (1989). *When anger hurts: Quieting the storm within*. Oakland, CA: New Harbinger Publications, Inc.

*Meichenbaum, D., and Turk, D.C. (1987). *Facilitating treatment adherence: A practitioner's guidebook*. NY: Plenum Press.

Paine, W.S. (Ed.). (1982). Job stress and burnout. Beverly Hills, CA: Sage Publications.

Patterson, G.R. (1975). *Families: Applications of social learning to family life*. Eugene, OR: Castalia Publishing.

Patterson, G.R. (1976). *Living with children: New methods for parents and teachers* (rev.). Champaign, IL: Research Press.

Peterson, C., and Bossio, L.M. (1991). *Health and optimism*. NY: The Free Press.

Sanders, H. (1993). *Body relaxed, mind at ease* (cassette tape: 90 minutes). Oakland, CA: New Harbinger Publications, Inc.

Selye, H. (1956). *The stress of life*. New York: McGraw-Hill.

Seyle, H. (1974). *Stress without distress*. New York: New American Library.

*Shapiro, A.K., and Morris, L.A. (1978). The placebo effect in medical and psychological therapies. In S.L. Garfield and A.E. Bergen (Eds.). *Handbook of psychotherapy and behavior change* (2nd ed.). New York: Wiley.

Skinner, B.F. (1979). *The shaping of a behaviorist*. NY: Knopf.

Sloane, H.N. (1992). *The good kid book: How to solve the 16 most common behavior problems*. Champaign, IL: Research Press.

Stevens, J.O. (1971). *Awareness: Exploring, experimenting, experiencing*. Moab, Utah: Real People Press.

Stutz, D.R., Feder, B., and Editors of Consumer Reports Books (1990). *The savvy patient: How to be an active participant in your medical care*. NY: Consumer Reports Books.

Tubesing, N.L., and Tubesing, D.H. (1990). *Structured exercises in stress management*. (vols. 1-4). Duluth, MN: Whole Person Press.

Williams, R.L., and Long, J.B. (1979). *Toward a self-managed life style* (2nd ed.). Boston: Houghton-Mifflin Company.

Zilberg, N.J., Weiss, D.S., and Horowitz, M.J. (1982). Impact of Event Scale: A Cross-Validation Study. *Journal of Consulting and Clinical Psychology, 50*, 407-414.

# Weight Control

*Baker, R.C., and Kirschenbaum, D.S. (1993). Self-monitoring may be necessary for successful weight control. *Behavior Therapy, 24*, 377-394.

Banting, W. (1863). *Letter on corpulence, addressed to the public (third edition)*. Kensington, England: Author. Reprinted in *Obesity Research* (1993) *1*, 153-161.

Barrett, S., and Editors of Consumer Reports. (1990). *Health schemes, scams, and frauds*. Mount Vernon, NY: Consumers Union.

Bennett, W., and Gurin J. (1982). *The dieter's dilemma*. New York: Basic Books.

Bennion, L.H., Bierman, E.L., and Ferguson, J.M. (1991). *Straight talk about weight control*. Fairfield, Ohio: Consumer Reports Books (telephone: 513/860/1178).

Brownell, K.D. (1990). *The LEARN program for weight control*. Dallas: The LEARN Education Center (telephone: 800/736/7323).

*Brownell, K.D., and Foreyt, J.P. (Eds.). (1986). *Handbook of eating disorders*. NY: Basic Books.

Colvin, R.H., and Olson, S.B. (1984). Winners revisited: An 18-month follow-up of our successful weight losers. *Addictive Behaviors, 9*, 305-306.

Colvin, R.H., and Olson, S.B. (1985). *Keeping it off.* NY: Simon & Schuster.

Coolidge, C. (1932). Persistence. From a speech given for the New York Life Insurance Company. According to Lawrence Wikander and Cynthia Bittinger of The Calvin Coolidge Memorial Foundation, Plymouth, Vermont 05056.

*Greenway, G. (1992). Non-prescription medications for weight control: A review. *American Journal of Clinical Nutrition, 55,* 203-205.

*Ikemi, Y., and Nakagawa, S. (1962). A psychosomatic study of contagious dermatitis. *Kyoshu Journal of Medical Science, 13,* 335-350.

*Johnson, W.G. (Ed.). (1987). *Advances in eating disorders, Vol. 1: Treating and preventing obesity.* Greenwich, CT: JAI Press.

*Kayman, S., Bruvold, W., and Stern, J.S. (1990). Maintenance and relapse after weight loss in women: Behavioral aspects. *American Journal of Clinical Nutrition, 52,* 800-807.

*Kirsch, I. (1990). *Changing expectations: A key to effective psychotherapy.* Pacific Grove, CA: Brooks/Cole.

*Kirschenbaum, D.S. (1987). Self-regulatory failure: A review with clinical implications. *Clinical Psychology Review, 7,* 77-104.

*Kirschenbaum, D.S. (1988). Treating adult obesity in 1988: Evolution of a modern program. *The Behavior Therapist, 11,* 3-6.

*Kirschenbaum, D.S. (1992). Elements of effective weight control programs: Implications for exercise and sport psychology. *Journal of Applied Sport Psychology, 4,* 77-93.

*Kirschenbaum, D.S., Fitzgibbon, M.L., Martino, S., Conviser, J.H., Rosendahl, E.H., and Laatsch, L. (1992). Stages of change in successful weight control: A clinically derived model. *Behavior Therapy, 23,* 623-635.

*Kirschenbaum, D.S., Johnson, W.G., and Stalonas, P.M. (1987). *Treating childhood and adolescent obesity.* NY: Pergamon Press.

*Kirschenbaum, D.S., and Tomarken, A.J. (1982). On facing the generalization problem: The study of self-regulatory failure. In P.C. Kendall (Ed.) *Advances in cognitive-behavioral research and therapy,* Vol. 1. New York: Academic Press.

*Marlatt, G.A., and Gordon, J.R. (Eds.). (1985). *Relapse prevention: Maintenance strategies in the treatment of addictive behaviors.* NY: Guilford Press.

National Institutes of Health. (1992). *Methods for voluntary weight loss and control: Technology Assessment Conference statement.* Bethesda, Maryland: NIH (available from: Office of Medical Applications of Research, NIH, Federal Building Room 618, Bethesda, MD 10892).

*Nelson, L.R., and Furst, M.L. (1972). An objective study of the effects of expectation on competitive performance. *Journal of Psychology, 81,* 69-72.

*Obesity and health.* Hettinger, North Dakota: Healthy Living Institute (telephone: 701/567/2845). This is an excellent newsletter that covers the current research on weight control and related issues.

*Perri, M.G., Nezu, A.M., and Viegener, B.J. (1992). *Improving the long-term management of obesity.* NY: John Wiley & Sons.

Rodin, J. (1992). *Body traps: Breaking the binds that keep you from feeling good about your body.* NY: William Morrow & Company.

Sandbek, T.J. (1993). *The deadly diet: Recovering from anorexia and bulimia* (2nd ed.). Oakland, CA: New Harbinger Publications, Inc.

*Smith, T.W., and Leon, A.S. (1992). *Coronary heart disease: A behavioral perspective.* Champaign, IL: Research Press.

*Stunkard, A.J. (Ed.). (1980). *Obesity.* Philadelphia: W.B. Saunders.

*Stunkard, A.J., and Wadden, T.A. (Eds.). (1993). *Obesity: Theory and therapy,* (2nd ed.). NY: Raven Press.

*Telch, C.F., and Agras, W.S. (1992). The effects of a very low calorie diet on binge eating. *Behavior Therapy, 24,* 177-193.

U.S. Department of Agriculture and U.S. Department of Health and Human Services. (1990). Nutrition and your health: Dietary guidelines for Americans (3rd Ed.). *Home and Garden Bulletin No. 232.* Washington, DC: Government Printing Office.

*Wadden, T.A., and Vanltallie, T.B. (Eds.). (1992). *Treatment of the seriously obese patient.* NY: Guilford Press.

Wasserstein, W. (1990). *Bachelor girls.* New York: Knopf.

*Weight Control Digest.* Dallas, TX: American Health Publishing Company (telephone: 800/736/7323). This is another excellent newsletter that summarizes many important research findings and ideas from experts on weight control.

# Other New Harbinger Self-Help Titles

*Coping With Schizophrenia: A Guide For Families*, $13.95
*Visualization for Change, Second Edition*, $13.95
*Postpartum Survival Guide*, $13.95
*Angry All The Time: An Emergency Guide to Anger Control*, $12.95
*Couple Skills: Making Your Relationship Work*, $13.95
*Handbook of Clinical Psychopharmacology for Therapists*, $39.95
*The Warrior's Journey Home: Healing Men, Healing the Planet*, $12.95
*Weight Loss Through Persistence*, $13.95
*Post-Traumatic Stress Disorder: A Complete Treatment Guide*, $39.95
*Stepfamily Realities: How to Overcome Difficulties and Have a Happy Family*, $11.95
*Leaving the Fold: A Guide for Former Fundamentalists and Others Leaving Their Religion*, $13.95
*Father-Son Healing: An Adult Son's Guide*, $12.95
*The Chemotherapy Survival Guide*, $11.95
*Your Family/Your Self: How to Analyze Your Family System*, $12.95
*Being a Man: A Guide to the New Masculinity*, $12.95
*The Deadly Diet, Second Edition: Recovering from Anorexia & Bulimia*, $11.95
*Last Touch: Preparing for a Parent's Death*, $11.95
*Consuming Passions: Help for Compulsive Shoppers*, $11.95
*Self-Esteem, Second Edition*, $13.95
*Depression & Anxiety Mangement: An audio tape for managing emotional problems*, $11.95
*I Can't Get Over It, A Handbook for Trauma Survivors*, $13.95
*Concerned Intervention, When Your Loved One Won't Quit Alcohol or Drugs*, $11.95
*Redefining Mr. Right*, $11.95
*Dying of Embarrassment: Help for Social Anxiety and Social Phobia*, $11.95
*The Depression Workbook: Living With Depression and Manic Depression*, $14.95
*Risk-Taking for Personal Growth: A Step-by-Step Workbook*, $11.95
*The Marriage Bed: Renewing Love, Friendship, Trust, and Romance*, $11.95
*Focal Group Psychotherapy: For Mental Health Professionals*, $44.95
*Hot Water Therapy: Save Your Back, Neck & Shoulders in 10 Minutes a Day* $11.95
*Older & Wiser: A Workbook for Coping With Aging*, $12.95
*Prisoners of Belief: Exposing & Changing Beliefs that Control Your Life*, $10.95
*Be Sick Well: A Healthy Approach to Chronic Illness*, $11.95
*Men & Grief: A Guide for Men Surviving the Death of a Loved One.*, $12.95
*When the Bough Breaks: A Helping Guide for Parents of Sexually Abused Childern*, $11.95
*Love Addiction: A Guide to Emotional Independence*, $12.95
*When Once Is Not Enough: Help for Obsessive Compulsives*, $11.95
*The New Three Minute Meditator*, $12.95
*Getting to Sleep*, $10.95
*The Relaxation & Stress Reduction Workbook, 3rd Edition*, $14.95
*Leader's Guide to the Relaxation & Stress Reduction Workbook*, $19.95
*Beyond Grief: A Guide for Recovering from the Death of a Loved One*, $10.95
*Thoughts & Feelings: The Art of Cognitive Stress Intervention*, $13.95
*Messages: The Communication Skills Book*, $12.95
*The Divorce Book*, $11.95
*Hypnosis for Change: A Manual of Proven Techniques, 2nd Edition*, $13.95
*The Chronic Pain Control Workbook*, $13.95
*Visualization for Change*, $12.95
*My Parent's Keeper: Adult Children of the Emotionally Disturbed*, $11.95
*When Anger Hurts*, $13.95
*Free of the Shadows: Recovering from Sexual Violence*, $12.95
*Lifetime Weight Control*, $11.95
*The Anxiety & Phobia Workbook*, $14.95
*Love and Renewal: A Couple's Guide to Commitment*, $12.95
*The Habit Control Workbook*, $12.95

Call **toll free, 1-800-748-6273**, to order. Have your Visa or Mastercard number ready. Or send a check for the titles you want to New Harbinger Publications, Inc., 5674 Shattuck Avenue, Oakland, CA 94609. Include $3.80 for the first book and 75¢ for each additional book, to cover shipping and handling. (California residents please include appropriate sales tax.) Allow four to six weeks for delivery.

*Prices subject to change without notice.*